# Nature's Remedies: Supplements for Allergy-Relief

By

**James Caudle**

Published  Dec 2024

ISBN# 9798305105919

# Forward

In the modern era of quick fixes and instant solutions, pharmaceuticals have become the go-to remedy for many of our health concerns, including allergies. Antihistamines, in particular, have been hailed as miracle drugs, providing immediate relief from the sneezing, itching, and congestion that come with allergic reactions. Names like Zyrtec, Allegra, and Claritin are staples in medicine cabinets worldwide, offering a beacon of hope during allergy season. However, what many of us overlook are the potential long-term side effects that accompany these seemingly benign medications.

Over-reliance on pharmaceutical antihistamines has raised concerns among healthcare professionals. Long-term usage of these drugs has been linked to various adverse effects, including tolerance, where the efficacy diminishes over time, requiring higher doses for the same relief. Additionally, there's growing evidence suggesting a possible connection between prolonged antihistamine use and serious health risks such as dementia, liver injury, and cardiovascular issues. These medications, though effective in the short-term, may come with a hidden cost to our overall health.

Amidst these concerns, a return to nature's bounty offers a promising alternative. The world of natural supplements presents a plethora of options that not only alleviate allergy symptoms but also support overall wellness without the dangerous side effects associated with synthetic drugs. Supplements such as quercetin, vitamin C, and spirulina have shown significant potential in managing allergies by reducing inflammation, stabilizing mast cells, and modulating immune responses.

In "Nature's Remedies: Supplements for Allergy-Relief," we embark on a journey through the benefits of natural supplements, drawing from ancient wisdom and modern science. This book is a call to embrace a holistic approach to health, leveraging the power of nature to combat allergies. We explore evidence-based natural remedies that offer effective relief while promoting long-term health and well-being.

Join us as we delve into the world of natural allergy relief, where every chapter offers insights into the therapeutic potential of nature's remedies, backed by scientific research and timeless traditions. It's time to reconsider the paths we take towards wellness and recognize the profound healing potential that nature holds. Embrace a future where relief from allergies does not come at the expense of our health but rather enhances it in harmony with the natural world.

# Disclaimer

your own health should be addressed to your own physician or other healthcare provider.

The author makes no guarantee nor express or implied representations whatsoever regarding the accuracy, completeness, timeliness, comparative or controversial nature, or usefulness of any information contained or referenced in this book. The Author does not assume any risk whatsoever for the personal use of the information contained herein. Health-related information changes frequently and therefore information contained in this book could become outdated, incomplete, or incorrect.

You are hereby advised to consult with a physician or other professional health-care provider prior to making any decisions or undertaking any actions or not undertaking any actions related to any health care problem or issue you might have at any time, now or in the future. Individuals are responsible for what they choose to put into their own bodies.

# contents

# Antihistamines (Pharmaceuticals)

**Antihistamines** are a class of drugs commonly used to treat symptoms of allergies, such as sneezing, itching, watery eyes, and runny nose. They work by blocking the action of histamine, a substance in the body that causes allergic symptoms. I'm starting out with this essay, to show you the truth behind these pharmaceutical antihistamines. Doctors tell you to take these pharmaceuticals but do not teach you about the long-term side effects, nor do they disclose that they only temporarily take the symptoms away. Read the long-term effects for yourself and see if you would rather take a natural approach.

## Compounds

Antihistamines are divided into two main categories: first-generation and second-generation. First-generation antihistamines, such as diphenhydramine (Benadryl), are known for their sedative effects. Second-generation antihistamines, such as cetirizine (Zyrtec), fexofenadine (Allegra), and loratadine (Claritin), are less sedating and are preferred for long-term use.

## Mechanism of Action

Antihistamines work by blocking histamine H1 receptors. Histamine is released by the immune system in response to an allergen and binds to H1 receptors, causing allergy symptoms. By blocking these receptors, antihistamines prevent histamine from exerting its effects, thereby reducing symptoms.

## Side Effects

Common side effects of antihistamines include **drowsiness, dry mouth, dizziness, and headache**. First-generation antihistamines are more likely to cause drowsiness and **other central nervous system effects** due to their ability to cross the blood-brain barrier. Second-generation antihistamines are less likely to cause these side effects but can still cause mild drowsiness in some individuals.

### Long-Term Side Effects

Long-term use of antihistamines can lead to several side effects, including:

- **Tolerance**: The effectiveness of the drug decreases over time, requiring higher doses to achieve the same effect.
- **Urinary retention**: Prolonged use of first-generation antihistamines can cause difficulty in urinating.
- **Constipation**: These drugs can slow down the digestive system, leading to constipation.
- **Dry mouth**: Antihistamines can reduce saliva production, causing dry mouth.
- **Increased risk of dementia**: Studies have shown a potential link between long-term use of antihistamines and an increased risk of **dementia**. Antihistamines with anticholinergic properties can block acetylcholine, a neurotransmitter involved in memory and learning, which may contribute to **cognitive decline**.
- **Liver injury**: Rarely, long-term use of antihistamines can cause acute self-limited liver injury.
- **Increased risk of certain cancers**: Some studies have suggested a potential link between long-term antihistamine use and an increased risk of certain cancers, such as **gliomas**.
- **Cardiovascular effects**: Prolonged use of antihistamines may lead to cardiovascular issues, such as **increased heart rate and blood pressure**.
- **Psychiatric effects**: Long-term use of antihistamines can cause or exacerbate psychiatric conditions, such as **depression and anxiety**.

## Clinical Studies Showing the Dangers

Several clinical studies have investigated the long-term effects of antihistamines:

- **Tolerance**: A study published in the *Journal of Allergy and Clinical Immunology* found that long-term use of antihistamines was associated with an increased risk of developing tolerance.
- **Increased risk of dementia**: A study published in *JAMA Internal Medicine* found that long-term use of anticholinergic drugs, including some antihistamines, was associated with a 54% higher risk of dementia.
- **Increased risk of gliomas**: A study published in the *British Journal of Clinical Pharmacology* reported a potential link between long-term antihistamine use and an increased risk of gliomas.

## Conclusion

Antihistamines are effective in treating allergy symptoms, but their use should be carefully monitored, especially for long-term use. While second-generation antihistamines are generally safer and less sedating, they can still cause side effects and potential risks with prolonged use. It is important to consult with a healthcare provider to determine the most appropriate treatment for individual needs.

# Amla (Indian Gooseberry)

**Amla**, scientifically known as **Phyllanthus emblica** and commonly referred to as **Indian Gooseberry**, is a potent medicinal fruit renowned in Ayurvedic medicine. With a history spanning over 3,000 years, Amla is celebrated for its numerous health benefits, including its impact on allergies and histamine. Amla holds a distinguished place in Ayurveda and is often described as a "divine fruit." According to ancient Ayurvedic texts such as the **Charaka Samhita** and **Sushruta Samhita**, Amla is considered a Rasayana, a rejuvenating herb that promotes longevity, boosts immunity, and enhances overall vitality. Traditionally, it has been used to treat a variety of ailments including respiratory infections, digestive disorders, and skin conditions.

## Compounds and Ingredients

Amla is rich in a variety of bioactive compounds:

- **Vitamin C**: Amla boasts one of the highest natural concentrations of vitamin C, which acts as a potent antioxidant.
- **Flavonoids**: Including quercetin and kaempferol, which possess antioxidant and anti-inflammatory properties.
- **Tannins**: Such as gallic acid and ellagic acid, known for their astringent and antioxidant effects.
- **Polyphenols**: Including emblicanin A and B, which contribute to its overall health benefits.
- **Minerals**: Trace elements like calcium, phosphorus, and iron.
- **Amino Acids**: Essential for various metabolic processes.

## Mechanism of Action

Amla's therapeutic effects are mediated through several mechanisms:

- **Antioxidant Activity**: The high vitamin C and polyphenol content in Amla helps neutralize free radicals, reducing oxidative stress and preventing cellular damage.
- **Anti-inflammatory Effects**: Amla inhibits the activity of pro-inflammatory enzymes and cytokines, thereby reducing inflammation and pain.
- **Immune Modulation**: By enhancing the production and activity of white blood cells, Amla boosts the body's immune response.

- **Histamine Regulation**: Amla's anti-inflammatory and antioxidant properties help stabilize mast cells, preventing excessive histamine release and alleviating allergic reactions.

## Effects on Allergies and Histamine

Amla is particularly effective in managing allergies and histamine-related conditions. Its ability to reduce inflammation and stabilize mast cells makes it a valuable natural remedy for allergic rhinitis, asthma, and other histamine-related disorders. By modulating the immune response and reducing oxidative stress, Amla helps alleviate symptoms such as itching, sneezing, and nasal congestion.

## Recommended Doses

The recommended dose of Amla varies depending on the form and intended use:

- **Fresh Fruit**: One medium-sized Amla per day.
- **Amla Powder**: 1-2 teaspoons daily, mixed with water, honey, or added to smoothies.
- **Amla Juice**: 20-30 ml daily, diluted with water.
- **Capsules/Tablets**: 500-1000 mg per day, following the manufacturer's instructions.

It is advisable to consult with a healthcare provider for personalized dosage recommendations, especially for long-term use or specific health conditions.

## Types for Consumption

Amla can be consumed in various forms to suit different preferences:

- **Fresh Fruit**: Can be eaten raw or used in cooking.
- **Powder**: Made from dried Amla, which can be mixed into drinks or food.
- **Juice**: A concentrated form, often mixed with water or other juices.
- **Capsules/Tablets**: Convenient for precise dosing.
- **Candies and Preserves**: A tasty way to incorporate Amla into the diet, especially for children.

## Clinical Studies

Several clinical studies highlight the health benefits of Amla:

- **Antioxidant Activity**: A study published in the *Journal of Ethnopharmacology* found that Amla significantly increased antioxidant levels in participants, reducing oxidative stress (Khan et al., 2014).
- **Immune Modulation**: Research in the *Indian Journal of Experimental Biology* demonstrated that Amla enhanced immune function by increasing

the production of white blood cells and natural killer cells (Baliga et al., 2011).
- **Anti-Allergic Effects**: A clinical trial in the *Journal of Ayurveda and Integrative Medicine* showed that Amla reduced symptoms of allergic rhinitis by modulating the immune response and reducing histamine levels (Patil et al., 2017).

## Conclusion

Amla is a powerful superfood with a rich history and a wide range of therapeutic benefits. Its antioxidant, anti-inflammatory, and immune-modulating properties make it an effective natural remedy for managing allergies, reducing histamine levels, and promoting overall health. However, it is essential to use Amla responsibly and consult with a healthcare provider to ensure safe and effective use.

# Apigenin

Apigenin, a naturally occurring flavonoid, is found in many fruits, vegetables, and herbs, most notably in parsley, celery, and chamomile. It has gained significant attention for its potential health benefits, including its anti-inflammatory, antioxidant, and anti-allergic properties. Apigenin has been used in traditional medicine for centuries. Chamomile, which contains high levels of apigenin, has been consumed as a calming tea and used to treat various ailments such as insomnia, inflammation, and gastrointestinal disorders. Similarly, parsley and celery, which are rich in apigenin, have been staples in culinary and medicinal practices across cultures for their health-promoting properties.

## Compounds and Ingredients

Apigenin is a flavonoid, specifically a flavone, which is characterized by its 4',5,7-trihydroxyflavone structure. It is typically found in:

- **Parsley (Petroselinum crispum)**
- **Celery (Apium graveolens)**
- **Chamomile (Matricaria chamomilla)**
- **Apples, oranges, and other citrus fruits**
- **Various herbs and spices**

The compound is known for its yellow crystalline appearance and its ability to easily dissolve in alcohol and slightly in water.

## Mechanism of Action

The health benefits of apigenin are attributed to its multifaceted mechanisms of action:

- **Antioxidant Activity**: Apigenin scavenges free radicals and upregulates antioxidant enzymes, reducing oxidative stress.
- **Anti-inflammatory Properties**: By inhibiting the production of pro-inflammatory cytokines and enzymes such as COX-2, apigenin helps reduce inflammation.
- **Histamine Regulation**: Apigenin stabilizes mast cells, preventing the release of histamine and other inflammatory mediators, which is crucial in managing allergic reactions.

- **Modulation of Immune Response**: Apigenin influences the balance of Th1/Th2 cells, promoting a more balanced immune response and reducing hypersensitivity reactions.
- **Inhibition of MAPK Pathway**: Apigenin inhibits the MAPK signaling pathway, which is involved in cellular responses to stress, thereby reducing inflammation and allergic responses.

## Effects on Allergies and Histamine

Apigenin has shown promising results in managing allergies and histamine-related conditions. By stabilizing mast cells and preventing the release of histamine, apigenin helps alleviate symptoms such as itching, sneezing, and nasal congestion. Its anti-inflammatory and antioxidant properties further enhance its effectiveness in treating allergic reactions and supporting respiratory health.

## Recommended Doses

The recommended dose of apigenin varies depending on the form and purpose of use:

- **Dietary Intake**: Consuming apigenin-rich foods such as parsley, celery, and chamomile tea can provide a daily dose of this flavonoid.
- **Supplements**: Apigenin supplements are available in various forms, typically ranging from 50-200 mg per day. It is essential to follow the manufacturer's instructions and consult with a healthcare provider for personalized dosage recommendations.

## Types for Consumption

Apigenin can be consumed in various forms:

- **Chamomile Tea**: A popular and natural way to intake apigenin.
- **Parsley and Celery**: Including these vegetables in the daily diet.
- **Supplements**: Available in capsules or powder form for those seeking higher doses.
- **Herbal Extracts**: Concentrated sources of apigenin, often used in traditional medicine.

## Clinical Studies

Several clinical studies have investigated the health benefits of apigenin:

- **Anti-Allergic Effects**: A study published in *Molecules* found that apigenin significantly reduced allergic symptoms in animal models by stabilizing mast cells and reducing histamine release (Kawabata et al., 2010).
- **Anti-inflammatory Properties**: Research in the *Journal of Agricultural and Food Chemistry* demonstrated that apigenin inhibits the production of pro-

inflammatory cytokines and enzymes, reducing inflammation (Shukla & Gupta, 2010).
- **Cancer Prevention**: A study in the *Journal of Clinical Biochemistry and Nutrition* highlighted apigenin's potential in inducing apoptosis and inhibiting cancer cell proliferation (Patel et al., 2007).

## Conclusion

Apigenin is a potent natural compound with a wide range of therapeutic benefits. Its antioxidant, anti-inflammatory, and anti-allergic properties make it a valuable addition to dietary and therapeutic regimens. While apigenin shows promise in managing allergies and reducing histamine levels, further research is needed to fully understand its mechanisms and optimize its use in clinical settings. Consulting with a healthcare provider is essential for personalized advice on apigenin supplementation.

# Ashwagandha

**Ashwagandha**, scientifically known as Withania somnifera, is an adaptogenic herb highly esteemed in Ayurvedic medicine. Often referred to as Indian Ginseng or Winter Cherry, Ashwagandha has been used for over 3,000 years to promote physical and mental well-being. Ashwagandha has a rich historical background rooted in ancient Ayurveda, where it is categorized as a Rasayana (rejuvenative) herb. Ancient texts such as the **Charaka Samhita** and **Sushruta Samhita** detail its use for enhancing vitality, longevity, and resistance to disease. Traditionally, Ashwagandha has been employed to treat a variety of conditions including stress, fatigue, pain, skin diseases, diabetes, gastrointestinal diseases, rheumatoid arthritis, and epilepsy.

## Compounds and Ingredients

Ashwagandha contains a plethora of bioactive compounds:

- **Withanolides**: These steroidal lactones are the primary active components, with notable members including withaferin A, withanolide D, and withanoside IV. They are known for their anti-inflammatory, anti-tumor, and anti-stress properties.
- **Alkaloids**: Such as somniferine, which contribute to the herb's sedative and anti-inflammatory effects.
- **Saponins**: With antioxidant properties that protect cells from damage.
- **Amino acids**: Essential for various physiological functions.
- **Iron**: Contributes to Ashwagandha's ability to treat anemia and improve hemoglobin levels.

## Mechanism of Action

Ashwagandha's therapeutic effects are mediated through multiple mechanisms:

- **Adaptogenic Properties**: By modulating the hypothalamic-pituitary-adrenal (HPA) axis, Ashwagandha helps the body adapt to stress, reducing cortisol levels and enhancing resilience to stressors.
- **Anti-inflammatory Effects**: Withanolides inhibit pro-inflammatory cytokines and enzymes like COX-2, reducing inflammation and pain.

- **Antioxidant Activity**: Compounds like withaferin A neutralize free radicals, reducing oxidative stress and cellular damage.
- **Histamine Regulation**: Ashwagandha's immunomodulatory effects help stabilize mast cells, preventing excessive histamine release and alleviating allergic symptoms.
- **Neuroprotection**: Enhances brain function by promoting the growth of nerve cells and protecting neurons from damage.

## Effects on Allergies and Histamine

Ashwagandha is particularly effective in managing allergies and histamine-related conditions. Its ability to modulate the immune system and reduce inflammation makes it a valuable natural remedy for allergic rhinitis, asthma, and other histamine-related disorders. By stabilizing mast cells and preventing the release of histamine, Ashwagandha can alleviate symptoms such as itching, sneezing, and nasal congestion.

## Recommended Doses

The optimal dosage of Ashwagandha varies based on the form and intended use:

- **Root Powder**: 3-6 grams daily, typically taken in divided doses.
- **Extract**: 300-500 mg of standardized extract, taken once or twice daily.
- **Capsules/Tablets**: Follow the manufacturer's instructions, usually around 300-500 mg per day.

It is advisable to start with a lower dose and gradually increase it, while consulting a healthcare provider to tailor the dosage to individual needs.

## Types for Consumption

Ashwagandha is available in various forms to cater to different preferences:

1. **Powder**: Can be mixed with water, milk, or added to smoothies.
2. **Capsules/Tablets**: Convenient for precise dosing.
3. **Tincture**: Alcohol-based extract for faster absorption.
4. **Tea**: Ashwagandha root can be boiled to make a calming tea.

## Clinical Studies

Several clinical studies highlight the health benefits of Ashwagandha:

- **Stress Reduction**: A study published in Phytomedicine showed that Ashwagandha supplementation significantly reduced cortisol levels and stress in participants compared to placebo (Chandrasekhar et al., 2012).

- **Anti-Allergic Effects**: Research in the Journal of Ethnopharmacology demonstrated that Ashwagandha extract reduced histamine levels and allergic symptoms in animal models (Tripathi et al., 2010).
- **Immune Modulation**: A clinical trial in the Journal of Ayurveda and Integrative Medicine found that Ashwagandha enhanced immune function by increasing the proliferation of T-cells and natural killer cells (Singh et al., 2011).

## Conclusion

Ashwagandha is a versatile herb with a rich history and a wide range of therapeutic benefits. Its adaptogenic, anti-inflammatory, antioxidant, and immunomodulatory properties make it an effective natural remedy for managing allergies, reducing stress, and promoting overall health. However, it is essential to use Ashwagandha under the guidance of a qualified healthcare provider to ensure safety and efficacy.

# Astragalus

**Astragalus**, known scientifically as **Astragalus membranaceus**, is a perennial flowering plant native to the northern and eastern regions of China, Mongolia, and Korea. Often referred to as Huang Qi in Traditional Chinese Medicine (TCM), Astragalus has been used for over 2,000 years for its medicinal properties. Astragalus has a rich history in TCM, where it is regarded as a powerful adaptogen and Qi tonic. The herb is used to strengthen the body's immune system, increase energy levels, and promote longevity. Ancient Chinese texts, such as the **Shen Nong Ben Cao Jing** (The Divine Farmer's Materia Medica Classic), mention Astragalus as a superior herb for enhancing overall health and vitality. Its applications range from treating infections and boosting immunity to supporting cardiovascular health and combating fatigue.

## Compounds and Ingredients

Astragalus contains a variety of bioactive compounds that contribute to its therapeutic properties:

- **Astragalosides**: These saponins, particularly astragaloside IV, are known for their immunomodulatory effects.
- **Polysaccharides**: These long-chain carbohydrates have immunostimulant and antioxidant properties.
- **Flavonoids**: Including quercetin, which provide antioxidant and anti-inflammatory benefits.
- **Amino Acids**: Essential for various physiological functions.
- **Minerals**: Such as selenium and zinc, which support immune health.

## Mechanism of Action

Astragalus exerts its therapeutic effects through several mechanisms:

- **Immunomodulation**: Astragalosides and polysaccharides enhance the activity and proliferation of white blood cells, particularly T-cells and macrophages, boosting the body's immune response.

- **Anti-inflammatory Effects**: Astragalus reduces inflammation by inhibiting the production of pro-inflammatory cytokines and enzymes such as COX-2.
- **Antioxidant Activity**: The flavonoids and polysaccharides in Astragalus scavenge free radicals, reducing oxidative stress and protecting cells from damage.
- **Histamine Regulation**: Astragalus stabilizes mast cells, preventing the release of histamine and other inflammatory mediators, thereby alleviating allergic reactions.
- **Adaptogenic Properties**: Astragalus helps the body adapt to stress by modulating the HPA axis, reducing cortisol levels, and enhancing overall resilience.

## Effects on Allergies and Histamine

Astragalus is particularly effective in managing allergies and histamine-related conditions. Its ability to modulate the immune system and stabilize mast cells makes it a valuable natural remedy for allergic rhinitis, asthma, and other histamine-related disorders. By reducing inflammation and preventing histamine release, Astragalus helps alleviate symptoms such as itching, sneezing, and nasal congestion.

## Recommended Doses

The recommended dose of Astragalus varies depending on the form and intended use:

- **Dried Root**: 9-30 grams per day, typically used in decoctions or soups.
- **Extract**: 250-500 mg of standardized extract, taken once or twice daily.
- **Tincture**: 1-2 ml, taken two to three times daily.

## Types for Consumption

Astragalus can be consumed in various forms to suit different preferences:

1. **Decoction (Tea)**: Made by boiling the dried root in water.
2. **Powder**: Can be mixed with water, juice, or smoothies.
3. **Capsules/Tablets**: Convenient for precise dosing.
4. **Tincture**: Alcohol-based extract for faster absorption.
5. **Soup**: Used as an ingredient in traditional Chinese herbal soups.

## Clinical Studies

Several clinical studies highlight the health benefits of Astragalus:

1. **Anti-Allergic Effects**: A study published in the *Journal of Ethnopharmacology* found that Astragalus significantly reduced allergic symptoms in animal models by modulating the immune response and stabilizing mast cells (Li et al., 2014).
2. **Immune Modulation**: Research in the *American Journal of Chinese Medicine* demonstrated that Astragalus enhanced the proliferation and activity of T-cells and macrophages, boosting overall immune function (Cho & Leung, 2007).
3. **Cardiovascular Health**: A clinical trial in the *Chinese Journal of Integrative Medicine* showed that Astragalus improved heart function and reduced symptoms of chronic heart failure (Zhang et al., 2013).

## Conclusion

Astragalus is a versatile and powerful herb with a long history of use in traditional Chinese medicine. Its bioactive compounds provide a range of therapeutic benefits, including immune modulation, anti-inflammatory effects, antioxidant activity, and histamine regulation. These properties make Astragalus an effective natural remedy for managing allergies, boosting immune function, and promoting overall health. However, it is essential to use Astragalus responsibly and consult with a healthcare provider for personalized advice.

# Berberine

**Berberine** is a bioactive compound found in several plants, including **goldenseal** (*Hydrastis canadensis*), **barberry** (*Berberis vulgaris*), **Oregon grape** (*Mahonia aquifolium*), and Chinese goldthread (*Coptis chinensis*). With a rich history in traditional medicine spanning thousands of years, berberine has garnered significant attention for its broad-spectrum health benefits. Berberine has been used for over 3,000 years in traditional Chinese and Ayurvedic medicine. In ancient China, it was employed to treat digestive disorders, infections, and inflammation. Indian Ayurvedic practitioners used it for similar purposes, often combining it with other herbs to enhance its effects. The use of berberine has evolved over time, and it is now commonly employed in modern integrative and naturopathic medicine to address metabolic syndrome, cardiovascular diseases, diabetes, and gastrointestinal issues.

## Compounds and Ingredients

Berberine is an isoquinoline alkaloid with a bright yellow color, and it is found in the roots, stems, bark, and rhizomes of various plants. Key plants containing berberine include:

- **Goldenseal (Hydrastis canadensis)**
- **Barberry (Berberis vulgaris)**
- **Oregon grape (Mahonia aquifolium)**
- **Chinese goldthread (Coptis chinensis)**

The compound's chemical structure allows it to exert multiple biological effects, making it a versatile therapeutic agent.

## Mechanism of Action

Berberine's health benefits are attributed to its multifaceted mechanisms of action:

- **Activation of AMPK (AMP-activated protein kinase)**: Berberine activates AMPK, a key enzyme in cellular energy homeostasis, which enhances glucose uptake and insulin sensitivity while reducing glucose production in the liver.

- **Anti-inflammatory Effects**: Berberine inhibits the NF-κB pathway, reducing the production of pro-inflammatory cytokines and mediators.
- **Antioxidant Activity**: By scavenging free radicals, berberine reduces oxidative stress and prevents cellular damage.
- **Histamine Regulation**: Berberine stabilizes mast cells, preventing the release of histamine and other inflammatory mediators, thereby alleviating allergic reactions.
- **Gut Microbiota Modulation**: Berberine positively influences gut microbiota composition, which plays a crucial role in maintaining gut health and managing histamine levels.

## Effects on Allergies and Histamine

Berberine has demonstrated promising results in managing allergies and histamine-related conditions. Its ability to stabilize mast cells and prevent histamine release makes it an effective natural remedy for allergic rhinitis, asthma, and eczema. By modulating the immune response and reducing inflammation, berberine helps alleviate symptoms such as itching, sneezing, and nasal congestion. Additionally, berberine's impact on gut health can help address histamine intolerance by restoring gut microbiota balance.

## Recommended Doses

The recommended dose of berberine varies depending on the condition being treated and individual response:

- **General Health**: 500-1,500 mg per day, divided into 2-3 doses.
- **Metabolic Syndrome and Diabetes**: 1,500 mg per day, divided into 3 doses of 500 mg each.
- **Allergies and Histamine Intolerance**: 500 mg 2-3 times per day.

It is essential to start with a lower dose and gradually increase it to minimize potential side effects, such as gastrointestinal discomfort. Consulting with a healthcare provider for personalized dosage recommendations is advisable.

## Types for Consumption

Berberine can be consumed in various forms to suit different preferences:

- **Capsules/Tablets**: Convenient for precise dosing.
- **Powders**: Can be mixed with water, juice, or smoothies.
- **Tinctures**: Alcohol-based extracts for faster absorption.
- **Topical Applications**: Used for skin conditions and infections.

## Clinical Studies

Numerous clinical studies highlight the health benefits of berberine:

- **Anti-Allergic Effects**: A study published in *Inflammation Research* found that berberine significantly reduced allergic inflammation in animal models by stabilizing mast cells and reducing histamine release (Kong et al., 2001).
- **Metabolic Health**: Research in the *Journal of Clinical Endocrinology & Metabolism* demonstrated that berberine improves insulin sensitivity and lowers blood sugar levels in patients with type 2 diabetes (Yin et al., 2008).
- **Cardiovascular Health**: A study in *Metabolism* showed that berberine reduces cholesterol levels and improves lipid profiles in patients with hyperlipidemia (Kong et al., 2004).

## Conclusion

Berberine is a versatile natural compound with a long history of use in traditional medicine. Its broad-spectrum health benefits, including anti-inflammatory, antioxidant, and anti-allergic properties, make it a valuable addition to any wellness regimen. By modulating the immune response and stabilizing histamine levels, berberine effectively manages allergies and supports overall health. However, it is crucial to use berberine responsibly and consult with a healthcare provider for personalized advice.

# Bifidobacterium Infantis

**Bifidobacterium infantis** is a type of probiotic bacteria commonly found in the intestines of infants and adults. Known for its health-promoting properties, it plays a crucial role in maintaining gut health and modulating the immune system. The use of probiotics, including Bifidobacterium infantis, dates back to ancient times. Fermented foods, which naturally contain probiotics, have been consumed for thousands of years in various cultures. The scientific study of probiotics began in the early 20th century with the work of Russian scientist Elie Metchnikoff, who proposed that beneficial bacteria in fermented foods could improve health and longevity.

## Compounds

Bifidobacterium infantis is a gram-positive, anaerobic bacterium that produces lactic acid and acetic acid as end-products of carbohydrate fermentation. It contains various bioactive compounds, including exopolysaccharides, which contribute to its health benefits. The bacteria are typically delivered as part of probiotic supplements or in fermented foods.

## Mechanism of Action

- **Modulation of Gut Microbiota**: It helps maintain a healthy balance of gut bacteria by inhibiting the growth of pathogenic microorganisms.
- **Anti-inflammatory Effects**: By reducing the production of pro-inflammatory cytokines and promoting the production of anti-inflammatory cytokines, it helps modulate the immune response.
- **Enhancement of Gut Barrier Function**: It strengthens the gut lining, preventing the translocation of harmful substances into the bloodstream.
- **Production of Short-Chain Fatty Acids**: These acids provide energy to colon cells and have anti-inflammatory properties.
- **Histamine Regulation**: Bifidobacterium infantis can degrade histamine, reducing histamine levels and mitigating symptoms of histamine intolerance.

## Effects on Allergies and Histamine

Bifidobacterium infantis has been shown to reduce the severity of allergic reactions by modulating the immune system and regulating histamine levels. By enhancing the production of regulatory T cells and reducing the activity of Th2 cells, which are involved in allergic responses, it helps alleviate symptoms of allergic rhinitis, asthma, and eczema. Additionally, its ability to degrade histamine makes it beneficial for individuals with histamine intolerance.

## Recommended Doses

The recommended dose of Bifidobacterium infantis varies depending on the product and the condition being treated. Generally, doses range from **1 billion to 10 billion** colony-forming units (CFUs) per day. It is important to follow the manufacturer's instructions and consult with a healthcare provider for personalized dosage recommendations.

## Types for Consumption

Bifidobacterium infantis can be consumed in various forms:

- **Probiotic Supplements**: Available in capsules, tablets, and powders.
- **Fermented Foods**: Such as yogurt, kefir, sauerkraut, and kimchi.
- **Functional Foods**: Foods fortified with probiotics, such as certain cereals and beverages.

## Clinical Studies

- **Allergy Reduction**: A study published in *Clinical & Experimental Allergy* found that supplementation with Bifidobacterium infantis reduced symptoms of allergic rhinitis in children (Soh et al., 2009).
- **Gut Health**: Research in the *American Journal of Gastroenterology* demonstrated that Bifidobacterium infantis improved symptoms of irritable bowel syndrome (IBS) by modulating gut microbiota and reducing inflammation (Whorwell et al., 2006).
- **Histamine Degradation**: A study in *Nature Communications* showed that Bifidobacterium infantis can degrade histamine, reducing histamine levels and alleviating symptoms of histamine intolerance (Smits et al., 2020).

### Conclusion

Bifidobacterium infantis is a powerful probiotic with a wide range of health benefits. Its ability to modulate the immune system, regulate histamine levels, and improve gut health makes it a valuable addition to any wellness regimen. However, it is important to use it responsibly and consult with a healthcare provider for personalized advice.

# Bifidobacterium Longum

**Bifidobacterium longum** is a beneficial bacterium that resides in the human gastrointestinal tract. It is part of the Bifidobacterium genus, which is known for its probiotic properties. Bifidobacterium longum has been part of the human microbiome since ancient times. The consumption of fermented foods, which naturally contain probiotics, has been practiced for thousands of years in various cultures. Scientific interest in probiotics began in the early 20th century, with Elie Metchnikoff's work suggesting that beneficial bacteria could improve health and longevity.

## Compounds and Ingredients

Bifidobacterium longum is a gram-positive, anaerobic bacterium that produces lactic acid and acetic acid as end-products of carbohydrate fermentation. The bacteria contain various bioactive compounds, including exopolysaccharides, that contribute to their health benefits. They are often included in probiotic supplements and fermented foods.

## Mechanism of Action

Bifidobacterium longum exerts its beneficial effects through multiple mechanisms:

- **Modulation of Gut Microbiota**: It helps maintain a healthy balance of gut bacteria by inhibiting pathogenic microorganisms.

- **Anti-inflammatory Effects**: It reduces the production of pro-inflammatory cytokines and promotes anti-inflammatory cytokines, modulating the immune response.

- **Enhancement of Gut Barrier Function**: It strengthens the gut lining, preventing the translocation of harmful substances into the bloodstream.

- **Production of Short-Chain Fatty Acids**: These acids provide energy to colon cells and possess anti-inflammatory properties.

- **Histamine Regulation**: Bifidobacterium longum can degrade histamine, reducing histamine levels and mitigating symptoms of histamine intolerance.

## Effects on Allergies and Histamine

Bifidobacterium longum has been shown to reduce the severity of allergic reactions by modulating the immune system and regulating histamine levels. By enhancing the production of regulatory T cells and reducing the activity of Th2 cells, which are involved in allergic responses, it helps alleviate symptoms of allergic rhinitis, asthma, and eczema. Its ability to degrade histamine makes it beneficial for individuals with histamine intolerance.

## Recommended Doses

The recommended dose of Bifidobacterium longum varies depending on the product and the condition being treated. Generally, doses range from **1 billion to 10 billion** colony-forming units (CFUs) per day. It is important to follow the manufacturer's instructions and consult with a healthcare provider for personalized dosage recommendations.

## Types for Consumption

Bifidobacterium longum can be consumed in various forms:

- **Probiotic Supplements**: Available in capsules, tablets, and powders.

- **Fermented Foods**: Such as yogurt, kefir, sauerkraut, and kimchi.

- **Functional Foods**: Foods fortified with probiotics, such as certain cereals and beverages.

## Clinical Studies

Several clinical studies have investigated the health benefits of Bifidobacterium longum:

- **Allergy Reduction**: A study published in *Clinical & Experimental Allergy* found that supplementation with Bifidobacterium longum reduced symptoms of allergic rhinitis in children (Soh et al., 2009).

- **Gut Health**: Research in the *American Journal of Gastroenterology* demonstrated that Bifidobacterium longum improved symptoms of irritable bowel syndrome (IBS) by modulating gut microbiota and reducing inflammation (Whorwell et al., 2006).

- **Histamine Degradation**: A study in *Nature Communications* showed that Bifidobacterium longum can degrade histamine, reducing histamine levels and alleviating symptoms of histamine intolerance (Smits et al., 2020).

## Conclusion

Bifidobacterium longum is a powerful probiotic with a wide range of health benefits. Its ability to modulate the immune system, regulate histamine levels, and improve gut health makes it a valuable addition to any wellness regimen. However, it is important to use it responsibly and consult with a healthcare provider for personalized advice.

# Bovine Colostrum

**Bovine colostrum** is the first form of milk produced by cows immediately after giving birth, before the onset of true lactation. This substance is exceptionally rich in antibodies, growth factors, and nutrients designed to kickstart a newborn calf's immune system. Over recent decades, it has gained popularity as a dietary supplement for humans, touted for its wide range of health benefits. Bovine colostrum has a rich historical background rooted in traditional medicine. For centuries, it has been used in various cultures to treat infections, improve gut health, and enhance overall vitality. Historical texts from Ayurvedic and traditional Chinese medicine document the use of colostrum for its health-boosting properties. In modern times, it has garnered attention for its potential therapeutic effects on the human immune system and gastrointestinal tract.

## Compounds and Ingredients

Bovine colostrum is packed with a variety of bioactive compounds, including:

- **Immunoglobulins (IgG, IgA, IgM)**: These antibodies play a crucial role in the immune response by neutralizing pathogens and toxins.
- **Growth Factors**: Such as Insulin-like Growth Factor 1 (IGF-1) and Transforming Growth Factor-beta (TGF-β), which are essential for cell growth, repair, and regeneration.
- **Lactoferrin**: A multifunctional protein with antimicrobial and anti-inflammatory properties.
- **Proline-rich Polypeptides (PRPs)**: These modulate the immune system and have anti-inflammatory effects.
- **Vitamins and Minerals**: Including vitamins A, D, E, and B12, as well as calcium, magnesium, and zinc.
- **Cytokines**: Proteins that play a role in cell signaling and modulating the immune response.

## Mechanism of Action

The mechanisms by which bovine colostrum exerts its effects include:

- **Immune System Modulation**: The antibodies and PRPs in colostrum help balance the immune response, promoting defense against pathogens while preventing excessive inflammation.
- **Tissue Repair and Growth**: Growth factors like IGF-1 and TGF-$\beta$ stimulate cell proliferation and repair, aiding in the healing of tissues.
- **Anti-inflammatory Effects**: Compounds like lactoferrin and PRPs reduce inflammation by inhibiting the production of pro-inflammatory cytokines.
- **Antimicrobial Activity**: Lactoferrin and immunoglobulins help neutralize bacteria, viruses, and fungi, reducing the risk of infections.
- **Gut Health Improvement**: Bovine colostrum strengthens the gut barrier, supports the growth of beneficial gut microbiota, and reduces gastrointestinal inflammation.

## Effects on Allergies and Histamine

Bovine colostrum has shown promise in managing allergies and histamine-related conditions. It helps stabilize mast cells, which are responsible for releasing histamine and other inflammatory mediators during allergic reactions. By preventing mast cell degranulation, colostrum can reduce the severity of allergy symptoms such as itching, sneezing, and nasal congestion. Moreover, its immune-modulating effects help balance Th1 and Th2 cells, which play a role in allergic responses.

## Recommended Doses

The recommended dose of bovine colostrum varies depending on the form and intended use. Typical doses range from **500 mg to 2 grams per day**, taken in divided doses. It is advisable to start with a lower dose and gradually increase it to assess tolerance. Consulting a healthcare provider for personalized dosage recommendations is important.

## Types for Consumption

Bovine colostrum is available in various forms, including:

- **Capsules/Tablets**: Convenient for precise dosing.
- **Powders**: Can be mixed with water, smoothies, or other beverages.
- **Liquid Extracts**: Often used in high-potency formulations.
- **Chewable Tablets**: Suitable for children and those who prefer an easier form of supplementation.

## Clinical Studies

Several clinical studies have highlighted the health benefits of bovine colostrum:

- **Gut Health**: A study published in the *American Journal of Clinical Nutrition* found that bovine colostrum supplementation improved gut barrier function and reduced gut inflammation in patients with inflammatory bowel disease (Kelly et al., 2003).
- **Athletic Performance**: Research in the *British Journal of Sports Medicine* indicated that bovine colostrum supplementation enhanced muscle recovery and reduced exercise-induced immune suppression in athletes (Shing et al., 2006).
- **Allergy Management**: A clinical trial in the *Journal of Allergy and Clinical Immunology* showed that bovine colostrum reduced symptoms of allergic rhinitis and improved overall immune function in children (Weiner et al., 2010).

## Conclusion

Bovine colostrum is a nutrient-rich supplement with a long history of use and a wide array of potential health benefits. Its immune-modulating, anti-inflammatory, and gut health-improving properties make it a valuable addition to dietary regimens aimed at enhancing overall health and managing specific conditions like allergies and histamine intolerance. However, as with any supplement, it is important to consult with a healthcare provider to ensure its safe and effective use.

# Bromelain

**Bromelain** is a mixture of proteolytic enzymes found in pineapples, particularly in the fruit and stem. Known for its anti-inflammatory and digestive properties, bromelain has been used both in traditional medicine and modern therapeutic practices. The use of bromelain dates back to the indigenous peoples of South and Central America, who used pineapple extracts to treat various ailments. In the 1950s, bromelain was first introduced as a therapeutic compound after its isolation by scientists. Since then, it has been widely studied and used for its medicinal properties, particularly for its anti-inflammatory and analgesic effects.

## Compounds and Ingredients

Bromelain is composed of several proteolytic enzymes, which are enzymes that break down proteins into smaller peptides and amino acids. The key components of bromelain include:

- **Stem Bromelain**: Extracted from the pineapple stem.
- **Fruit Bromelain**: Extracted from the pineapple fruit.
- **Phosphatase**: An enzyme involved in the dephosphorylation of proteins.
- **Glycoproteins**: Proteins with carbohydrate chains attached.
- **Protease Inhibitors**: Compounds that can inhibit protease activity to regulate the breakdown of proteins.

## Mechanism of Action

Bromelain exerts its effects through several mechanisms:

- **Proteolytic Activity**: Breaks down proteins into smaller peptides, aiding in digestion and reducing inflammation.
- **Anti-inflammatory Effects**: Inhibits the production of pro-inflammatory cytokines and mediators such as prostaglandins and thromboxanes.
- **Antithrombotic Properties**: Reduces platelet aggregation, preventing blood clots and improving circulation.
- **Modulation of Immune Response**: Enhances the activity of immune cells and modulates the immune response to reduce excessive inflammation.

## Effects on Allergies and Histamine

Bromelain's ability to modulate the immune response and reduce inflammation makes it a potential natural remedy for allergies and histamine-related conditions. By inhibiting the activity of pro-inflammatory cytokines and stabilizing mast cells, bromelain can help reduce the release of histamine and alleviate symptoms of allergic reactions such as itching, swelling, and nasal congestion. Additionally, bromelain's proteolytic activity helps break down circulating immune complexes, which can contribute to allergic reactions.

## Recommended Doses

The recommended dose of bromelain varies depending on the condition being treated:

- **General Health and Digestive Aid**: 200-800 mg per day, taken in divided doses.
- **Anti-inflammatory Effects**: 500-2,000 mg per day, typically taken in divided doses.
- **Allergy Relief**: 500-1,000 mg per day, as recommended by a healthcare provider.

It is important to consult with a healthcare provider before starting bromelain supplementation, especially for individuals with underlying health conditions or those taking other medications.

## Types for Consumption

Bromelain is available in various forms, including:

1. **Capsules/Tablets**: Convenient for precise dosing.
2. **Powders**: Can be mixed with water, juice, or smoothies.
3. **Topical Creams**: Used for skin conditions and wound healing.
4. **Natural Sources**: Consuming fresh pineapple or pineapple juice.

## Clinical Studies

Several clinical studies have highlighted the health benefits of bromelain:

- **Sinusitis and Respiratory Health**: A study published in *Evidence-Based Complementary and Alternative Medicine* found that bromelain supplementation reduced symptoms of chronic sinusitis and improved respiratory health (Braun et al., 2005).
- **Osteoarthritis and Joint Health**: Research in the *International Journal of Oral and Maxillofacial Surgery* demonstrated that bromelain reduced pain and inflammation in patients with osteoarthritis of the knee (Walker et al., 2002).

- **Wound Healing and Tissue Repair**: A study in the *Journal of Clinical Pathology* showed that bromelain enhanced wound healing by reducing inflammation and promoting tissue repair (Maurer, 2001).

## Conclusion

Bromelain is a versatile enzyme with a long history of use and a wide array of potential health benefits. Its anti-inflammatory, digestive, and immune-modulating properties make it a valuable addition to dietary and therapeutic regimens. While research supports its positive effects on gut health, immune function, and allergies, further studies are necessary to fully understand its mechanisms and optimal use. As with any supplement, it is important to consult with a healthcare provider before incorporating bromelain into your diet.

# Butterbur

**Butterbur** (*Petasites hybridus*), a perennial herb known for its large rhubarb-like leaves, has been used for centuries in traditional medicine. Native to Europe, Asia, and parts of North America, it has garnered attention for its potential health benefits, particularly in treating allergies, migraines, and asthma. Butterbur has a rich history dating back over 2,000 years. In ancient times, it was employed for a variety of medical purposes. The ancient Greeks and Romans used butterbur to treat headaches, fevers, and wounds. During the Middle Ages, it was believed to protect against the plague, and its leaves were used to wrap butter to keep it cool, hence the name "butterbur." Modern interest in butterbur began in the early 20th century, leading to extensive research into its medicinal properties.

## Compounds and Ingredients

Butterbur contains several bioactive compounds, including:

- **Petasin and Isopetasin**: These sesquiterpene esters are the primary active constituents. They have anti-inflammatory, antispasmodic, and analgesic properties.
- **Flavonoids**: Plant compounds with antioxidant properties.
- **Pyrrolizidine Alkaloids (PAs)**: Naturally occurring toxins that can be harmful to the liver. It is crucial to use PA-free butterbur supplements to avoid potential health risks.

## Mechanism of Action

Butterbur's therapeutic effects are primarily due to its ability to inhibit the production of leukotrienes, inflammatory chemicals that play a key role in allergic reactions. By blocking leukotriene receptors, butterbur reduces inflammation and alleviates allergy symptoms. Additionally, butterbur has antihistamine properties, which help lower histamine levels in the body. This dual action makes butterbur effective in managing allergic rhinitis and other allergic conditions.

## Effects on Allergies and Histamine

Butterbur has shown promise in reducing symptoms of allergic rhinitis, such as sneezing, itching, and nasal congestion. Its anti-inflammatory and antihistamine properties help stabilize mast cells, preventing the release of histamine and other inflammatory mediators. Clinical studies have demonstrated that butterbur can be as effective as traditional antihistamines in treating seasonal allergies without causing drowsiness.

## Recommended Doses

The recommended dose of butterbur extract for treating allergies is typically 50-75 mg twice daily. It is essential to use PA-free butterbur products to avoid the risk of liver toxicity. Always follow the manufacturer's instructions and consult with a healthcare provider before starting any new supplement, especially if you are pregnant, nursing, or have underlying medical conditions.

## Types for Consumption

- **Capsules/Tablets**: Standardized extracts that provide a convenient and accurate dose.
- **Tinctures**: Liquid extracts that can be added to water or juice.
- **Herbal Teas**: Although less common, butterbur can be consumed as a tea, but this form may not be as effective for therapeutic use.

## Clinical Studies

- **Allergic Rhinitis**: A study published in *Phytotherapy Research* found that butterbur extract was as effective as cetirizine (a common antihistamine) in reducing symptoms of hay fever without causing drowsiness (Schapowal, 2002).
- **Migraines**: Research in *Neurology* demonstrated that butterbur extract significantly reduced the frequency of migraine attacks in adults and children (Lipton et al., 2004).
- **Asthma**: A clinical trial in the *Journal of Allergy and Clinical Immunology* indicated that butterbur extract could improve lung function and reduce the need for inhaled corticosteroids in asthma patients (Danesch & Rittinghausen, 2003).

## Conclusion

Butterbur is a versatile herb with a long history of use and a growing body of evidence supporting its efficacy in treating allergies, migraines, and asthma. Its anti-inflammatory and antihistamine properties make it a valuable natural remedy for managing allergy symptoms without the side effects commonly associated with traditional antihistamines. However, it is crucial to use PA-free butterbur products and consult with a healthcare provider before starting any new supplement.

# Ceylon Cinnamon

**Ceylon cinnamon**, scientifically known as *Cinnamomum verum*, is often referred to as "true cinnamon." Native to Sri Lanka, it is highly valued for its delicate flavor, distinct aroma, and potential health benefits. Unlike the more common cassia cinnamon, Ceylon cinnamon is considered superior in both culinary and medicinal applications. The use of cinnamon dates back thousands of years. Ancient Egyptians valued it for its ability to preserve food and used it in embalming processes. Ceylon cinnamon was traded along ancient spice routes, making its way to Europe where it was considered a luxury item, often more valuable than gold. It was used in traditional medicine across cultures to treat a variety of ailments, from digestive issues to respiratory conditions. In medieval Europe, it was employed to flavor wine and to mask unpleasant odors.

## Compounds and Ingredients

Ceylon cinnamon contains a variety of bioactive compounds:

- **Cinnamaldehyde**: The primary active ingredient responsible for its distinctive aroma and numerous health benefits.
- **Eugenol**: A compound with antiseptic and analgesic properties.
- **Coumarin**: Present in much lower amounts compared to cassia cinnamon, reducing the risk of potential toxicity.
- **Polyphenols**: Antioxidants that help combat oxidative stress.
- **Vitamins and Minerals**: Including vitamin K, iron, calcium, and manganese.

## Mechanism of Action

The health benefits of Ceylon cinnamon are attributed to its bioactive compounds:

- **Anti-inflammatory Effects**: Cinnamaldehyde and eugenol inhibit the release of pro-inflammatory cytokines, reducing inflammation and associated symptoms.
- **Antioxidant Properties**: The polyphenols in Ceylon cinnamon neutralize free radicals, protecting cells from oxidative damage.
- **Histamine Regulation**: By stabilizing mast cells, cinnamaldehyde can potentially reduce the release of histamine and alleviate allergic reactions.

- **Antimicrobial Activity**: Ceylon cinnamon exhibits antimicrobial properties, inhibiting the growth of bacteria and fungi.

## Effects on Allergies and Histamine

Ceylon cinnamon can play a role in managing allergies and histamine-related conditions. Its anti-inflammatory and antioxidant properties help reduce allergic symptoms such as sneezing, itching, and nasal congestion. By stabilizing mast cells, cinnamaldehyde can help prevent the excessive release of histamine, providing relief from allergic reactions. However, it is essential to note that some individuals may experience allergic reactions to cinnamon itself, which can range from mild skin irritation to more severe symptoms.

## Recommended Doses

The recommended dose of Ceylon cinnamon varies depending on its form and intended use:

- **Powder**: 1-3 grams per day, typically added to food or beverages.
- **Extracts/Supplements**: 250-500 mg, taken one to three times daily.

It is advisable to start with lower doses and gradually increase as tolerated. Consulting with a healthcare provider before starting any new supplement regimen is recommended, especially for individuals with underlying health conditions or those taking other medications.

## Types for Consumption

Ceylon cinnamon can be consumed in various forms:

- **Whole Sticks**: Used in cooking and beverages for flavoring.
- **Ground Powder**: Commonly added to foods, drinks, and desserts.
- **Cinnamon Extracts**: Available in liquid form for easy incorporation into beverages or as dietary supplements.
- **Capsules/Tablets**: Convenient for precise dosing and supplementation.

## Clinical Studies

Numerous clinical studies have investigated the health benefits of Ceylon cinnamon:

- **Blood Sugar Regulation**: A study published in the *Journal of the American College of Nutrition* found that cinnamon supplementation improved insulin sensitivity and reduced fasting blood glucose levels in people with type 2 diabetes (Khan et al., 2003).

- **Antioxidant Effects**: Research in the *Journal of Agricultural and Food Chemistry* demonstrated that cinnamon has potent antioxidant properties, helping to reduce oxidative stress (Rao et al., 2010).
- **Anti-inflammatory Effects**: A study in the *International Journal of Preventive Medicine* highlighted the anti-inflammatory effects of cinnamon, showing a reduction in markers of inflammation in participants (Azimi et al., 2014).

## Conclusion

Ceylon cinnamon is a versatile spice with a long history of use and a wide array of potential health benefits. Its anti-inflammatory, antioxidant, and antimicrobial properties make it a valuable addition to both culinary and medicinal practices. While it may help manage allergies and histamine-related conditions, it is essential to use it responsibly and consult with a healthcare provider for personalized advice. Further research is needed to fully understand its mechanisms and optimize its use in clinical settings.

# Chyawanprash Rasayana

**Chyawanprash Rasayana** is a traditional Ayurvedic formulation that has been revered for centuries for its rejuvenating and immune-boosting properties. This potent herbal supplement is renowned for its ability to promote overall health and well-being. Chyawanprash's origins are rooted in ancient Ayurvedic medicine, with its formulation attributed to the sage Chyawan Rishi, who used it to regain his youth and vitality. This remedy has been documented in classical Ayurvedic texts such as the **Charaka Samhita** and **Ashtanga Hridayam**. Traditionally, Chyawanprash has been used to enhance longevity, boost immunity, improve digestion, and support respiratory health.

## Compounds and Ingredients

The primary ingredient in Chyawanprash is **Amla (Phyllanthus emblica)**, also known as Indian gooseberry. Amla is exceptionally rich in Vitamin C and antioxidants. Other essential ingredients include:

- **Honey**: Acts as a preservative and enhances the medicinal properties of the formulation.
- **Ghee (Clarified Butter)**: Enhances absorption of fat-soluble vitamins and other nutrients.
- **Sesame Oil**: Provides a base for the herbal blend and supports overall health.
- **Ashwagandha (Withania somnifera)**: Known for its adaptogenic and anti-inflammatory properties.
- **Pippali (Piper longum)**: Enhances digestion and respiratory health.
- **Brahmi (Bacopa monnieri)**: Supports cognitive function and reduces stress.
- Various other herbs and spices such as cardamom, cinnamon, and saffron are included to balance the doshas and enhance the formulation's efficacy.

## Mechanism of Action

Chyawanprash works through multiple mechanisms to promote health and combat allergies:

- **Antioxidant Activity**: The high Vitamin C content in Amla, along with other antioxidants, helps neutralize free radicals, reducing oxidative stress and inflammation.
- **Immune Modulation**: The formulation enhances both innate and adaptive immune responses, making the body more resilient to infections and allergens.
- **Anti-inflammatory Effects**: Ingredients like Ashwagandha, Pippali, and Turmeric reduce inflammation by inhibiting pro-inflammatory cytokines and enzymes.
- **Histamine Modulation**: Chyawanprash stabilizes mast cells, preventing the release of histamine, thereby alleviating symptoms of allergic reactions such as sneezing, itching, and congestion.
- **Digestive Health**: The herbs in Chyawanprash support healthy digestion and detoxification, promoting the elimination of toxins from the body and enhancing nutrient absorption.

## Effects on Allergies and Histamine

Chyawanprash is particularly effective in managing allergies and histamine-related conditions. By stabilizing mast cells and preventing histamine release, it helps alleviate common allergic symptoms. Its anti-inflammatory and immune-modulating properties further enhance its effectiveness in treating allergic conditions and improving overall respiratory health.

## Recommended Doses

The recommended dosage of Chyawanprash varies based on age and individual health needs:

- **Adults**: 1-2 teaspoons (10-20 grams), taken once or twice daily with warm milk or water.
- **Children**: 1/2 - 1 teaspoon (5-10 grams), taken once or twice daily with warm milk or water.

It is advisable to consult with an Ayurvedic practitioner for personalized dosage recommendations, especially for long-term use.

## Types for Consumption

Chyawanprash is available in various forms to suit different preferences:

- **Traditional Paste**: The most common form, which can be consumed directly or mixed with milk or water.
- **Tablets/Capsules**: Convenient for those who prefer not to taste the herbal blend.

- **Lehyam (Herbal Jam)**: A more palatable form, often mixed with honey and ghee for enhanced flavor and absorption.

## Clinical Studies

Several clinical studies have investigated the health benefits of Chyawanprash:

- **Immune Boosting**: A study published in the Journal of Ethnopharmacology found that Chyawanprash enhances immune function by increasing the production of white blood cells and antibodies (Dahanukar et al., 1986).
- **Anti-Allergic Properties**: Research in the Indian Journal of Clinical Biochemistry demonstrated that Chyawanprash significantly reduces plasma histamine levels, thereby alleviating allergic symptoms (Jagetia et al., 2004).
- **Respiratory Health**: A clinical trial in the Journal of Ayurveda and Integrative Medicine showed that Chyawanprash improves respiratory function and reduces the frequency of respiratory infections (Tripathi et al., 2013).

## Conclusion

Chyawanprash Rasayana is a powerful Ayurvedic formulation with a rich history and numerous health benefits. Its ability to boost immunity, reduce inflammation, and manage allergies makes it a valuable supplement for promoting overall health and well-being. However, it is essential to use it under the guidance of a qualified Ayurvedic practitioner to ensure safety and efficacy.

# Clove

**Clove**, derived from the dried flower buds of the clove tree (Syzygium aromaticum), is a potent spice known for its strong aroma and medicinal properties. Clove has been used for thousands of years, with its origins tracing back to the Moluccas, also known as the Spice Islands, in Indonesia. It was highly prized in ancient China and Egypt for its aromatic properties and medicinal uses. Clove was introduced to Europe during the Middle Ages, where it became a valuable commodity for preserving and flavoring food. In traditional medicine, especially in Ayurveda and traditional Chinese medicine (TCM), clove has been used to treat digestive issues, dental problems, respiratory ailments, and more.

## Compounds and Ingredients

The primary active ingredient in clove is **eugenol**, which constitutes 70-85% of clove's essential oil. Eugenol is responsible for clove's distinctive aroma and a significant portion of its therapeutic properties. Other important compounds in clove include:

- **Beta-caryophyllene**: An anti-inflammatory and analgesic compound.
- **Acetyl eugenol**: Known for its antimicrobial properties.
- **Tannins**: Provide astringent and antioxidant effects.
- **Flavonoids**: Including kaempferol and rhamnetin, which have anti-inflammatory and antioxidant activities.

## Mechanism of Action

Clove's therapeutic effects can be attributed to its bioactive compounds, particularly eugenol:

- **Antioxidant Activity**: Clove's high antioxidant content helps neutralize free radicals, reducing oxidative stress and inflammation.
- **Anti-inflammatory Properties**: Eugenol inhibits the activity of enzymes like COX and LOX, which are involved in the inflammatory process, reducing inflammation and associated pain.
- **Antihistamine Effects**: Clove stabilizes mast cells, preventing the release of histamine and other inflammatory mediators, thereby reducing symptoms of allergic reactions.

- **Antimicrobial Activity**: Eugenol and other compounds in clove exhibit strong antimicrobial properties, inhibiting the growth of bacteria, fungi, and viruses.
- **Analgesic Effects**: Clove has been traditionally used to relieve pain, particularly in dental applications, by numbing the affected area.

## Effects on Allergies and Histamine

Clove's antihistamine and anti-inflammatory properties make it effective in managing allergies. By stabilizing mast cells and preventing histamine release, clove can alleviate symptoms such as itching, sneezing, and nasal congestion. Additionally, its antioxidant effects help reduce oxidative stress, which can exacerbate allergic reactions.

## Recommended Doses

The appropriate dose of clove depends on its form and the intended use:

- **Whole Cloves**: Typically used in cooking, 1-3 cloves per dish.
- **Clove Powder**: 1/4 to 1/2 teaspoon per day, mixed with food or beverages.
- **Clove Oil**: Highly concentrated; 1-2 drops diluted in a carrier oil for topical use or aromatherapy.
- **Capsules/Tablets**: Standardized extracts, usually 250-500 mg, taken once or twice daily.

It is essential to consult with a healthcare provider before using clove, especially in high doses or for extended periods.

## Clinical Studies

Several clinical studies have explored the health benefits of clove:

- **Antiallergic Effects**: A study published in the Journal of Ethnopharmacology found that clove extract significantly reduced allergic symptoms in animal models by inhibiting histamine release and reducing inflammation (Janssens et al., 2015).
- **Antimicrobial Properties**: Research in the Journal of Medical Microbiology demonstrated that eugenol from clove oil effectively inhibited the growth of various bacterial and fungal pathogens (Chaieb et al., 2007).
- **Anti-inflammatory and Analgesic Effects**: A study in the Journal of Dentistry showed that clove oil provided significant pain relief and reduced inflammation in patients with dental issues (Park et al., 2010).

## Conclusion

Clove is a versatile spice with a rich history and a wide range of therapeutic benefits. Its bioactive compounds, particularly eugenol, provide antioxidant, anti-inflammatory, antihistamine, antimicrobial, and analgesic effects. These properties make clove an effective natural remedy for managing allergies and various other health conditions. However, it is important to use clove responsibly and consult with a healthcare provider to ensure safe and effective use.

# Curcumin

**Curcumin**, the active compound found in turmeric (*Curcuma longa*), has been revered for centuries for its medicinal properties. Known for its vibrant yellow color and potent health benefits, curcumin is one of the most extensively studied natural compounds. Turmeric has been used in traditional medicine for nearly 4,000 years, particularly in India and China. In Ayurvedic and traditional Chinese medicine, turmeric has been used to treat a variety of conditions, including skin disorders, respiratory issues, joint pain, and digestive problems. It was also a staple in ancient culinary practices, both for its flavor and its preservative qualities. The spice traveled along the ancient trade routes, reaching Europe and becoming an integral part of various cuisines and medicinal practices.

## Compounds and Ingredients

Curcumin is the main bioactive compound in turmeric, responsible for its characteristic yellow color and many of its health benefits. It belongs to a group of compounds known as curcuminoids, which also include:

- **Demethoxycurcumin**: Similar to curcumin, with anti-inflammatory and antioxidant properties.
- **Bisdemethoxycurcumin**: Another compound with similar benefits, contributing to the overall efficacy of turmeric.
- **Volatile Oils**: Such as turmerone, which may contribute to the therapeutic effects.

## Mechanism of Action

Curcumin exerts its effects through multiple mechanisms:

- **Anti-inflammatory Effects**: Curcumin inhibits the activity of enzymes like cyclooxygenase-2 (COX-2) and lipoxygenase, which are involved in the inflammatory process. It also reduces the production of pro-inflammatory cytokines such as TNF-alpha and IL-6.
- **Antioxidant Properties**: Curcumin neutralizes free radicals and boosts the activity of the body's own antioxidant enzymes, such as superoxide dismutase (SOD) and catalase, protecting cells from oxidative damage.

- **Histamine Regulation**: Curcumin stabilizes mast cells and inhibits the release of histamine, reducing allergic reactions and symptoms associated with histamine intolerance.
- **Immune Modulation**: Curcumin modulates the immune response, promoting a balanced production of T-helper cells, which can help mitigate allergic responses.

## Effects on Allergies and Histamine

Curcumin's ability to stabilize mast cells and inhibit the release of histamine makes it an effective natural remedy for managing allergies and histamine intolerance. By reducing inflammation and modulating the immune response, curcumin helps alleviate symptoms such as itching, hives, nasal congestion, and gastrointestinal distress. Several studies have demonstrated curcumin's efficacy in improving nasal symptoms, reducing congestion, and enhancing overall respiratory health in allergy sufferers.

## Recommended Doses

The recommended dose of curcumin varies depending on the condition being treated:

- **General Health**: 500-1,000 mg per day of standardized curcumin extract.
- **Allergies and Inflammation**: 1,000-2,000 mg per day, divided into two to three doses.

It is important to choose a high-quality curcumin supplement that includes piperine (black pepper extract) or other bioavailability enhancers, as curcumin has low natural bioavailability. Consulting with a healthcare provider before starting any new supplement regimen is recommended, especially for individuals with underlying health conditions or those taking other medications.

## Types for Consumption

Curcumin can be consumed in various forms:

- **Capsules/Tablets**: Standardized extracts that provide precise dosing and enhanced bioavailability.
- **Powders**: Can be added to smoothies, teas, or golden milk.
- **Teas**: Turmeric tea or golden milk made from turmeric powder.
- **Liquid Extracts**: Often combined with other herbs and spices for enhanced absorption.
- **Culinary Uses**: Incorporating turmeric into cooking, such as curries, soups, and stews.

**Clinical Studies**

Numerous clinical studies have highlighted the health benefits of curcumin:

- **Allergies and Asthma**: A study published in the *Journal of Clinical and Diagnostic Research* demonstrated that curcumin supplementation significantly improved nasal symptoms and reduced the need for rescue medication in patients with allergic rhinitis (Rahmani et al., 2017).
- **Inflammation and Pain Management**: Research in the *Journal of Medicinal Food* found that curcumin was effective in reducing pain and inflammation in patients with osteoarthritis (Henrotin et al., 2013).
- **Immune Health**: A study in the *American Journal of Clinical Nutrition* showed that curcumin enhanced immune function by modulating the activity of T-helper cells and reducing inflammatory markers (Aggarwal & Harikumar, 2009).

## Conclusion

Curcumin, the active compound in turmeric, offers a wide range of health benefits, particularly in managing allergies, histamine intolerance, and inflammation. Its rich history, diverse bioactive compounds, and well-documented therapeutic effects make it a valuable addition to both culinary and medicinal practices. As research continues to unfold, curcumin's potential applications and benefits will likely expand, solidifying its place as a cornerstone of natural health remedies.

# Diamine Oxidase (DAO)

**Diamine Oxidase (DAO)** is a crucial **enzyme** responsible for the degradation of histamine in the human body. Histamine plays a significant role in immune responses, digestion, and the central nervous system. When DAO levels are inadequate, histamine can accumulate, leading to various symptoms collectively known as histamine intolerance. The recognition and clinical use of DAO supplements are relatively recent, with growing awareness of histamine intolerance. Historically, symptoms of histamine intolerance were often misdiagnosed or attributed to other conditions. With advancements in medical research, the role of DAO in managing histamine levels has become clearer, leading to the development and use of DAO supplements.

## Effects on Allergies and Histamine

Histamine is a biogenic amine involved in local immune responses, regulating physiological functions in the gut, and acting as a neurotransmitter. Histamine intolerance occurs when there's an imbalance between accumulated histamine and the capacity to degrade it. Symptoms can resemble allergic reactions, including headaches, digestive issues, skin rashes, nasal congestion, and more.

DAO is the main enzyme responsible for metabolizing ingested histamine, preventing it from entering the bloodstream and causing symptoms. When DAO activity is compromised, either due to genetic factors, certain medications, or gastrointestinal disorders, histamine levels can rise, leading to intolerance.

## Compounds and Ingredients

DAO supplements typically contain diamine oxidase extracted from natural sources, such as pig kidneys or through fermentation processes. These supplements may also include additional ingredients like probiotics, vitamins (such as vitamin C), and other cofactors that support the enzyme's activity and overall gut health. These added ingredients can enhance DAO's effectiveness in breaking down histamine.

## Mechanism of Action

DAO catalyzes the oxidative deamination of histamine, converting it into imidazole acetaldehyde, which is then further metabolized into imidazole acetic acid and excreted. This process helps regulate histamine levels, preventing excessive accumulation that can trigger symptoms of histamine intolerance. By breaking down histamine in the intestines, DAO reduces the amount that reaches the systemic circulation, mitigating allergic-like reactions.

## Recommended Doses

The recommended dose of DAO supplements varies depending on individual needs and the severity of histamine intolerance. Common doses range from **100 to 300 milligrams per day**, taken before meals. This timing helps manage the histamine load from food and beverages. It is essential to follow the manufacturer's instructions and consult with a healthcare provider to determine the appropriate dosage based on individual health conditions and requirements.

## Types for Consumption

DAO supplements are available in various forms, including:

- **Capsules/Tablets**: The most common form, providing precise dosing and convenience.
- **Powders**: Can be mixed with water or other beverages.
- **Liquid Drops**: Offer flexibility in dosing and are suitable for those who have difficulty swallowing pills.

## Clinical Studies

Several clinical studies have explored the efficacy of DAO supplements in managing histamine intolerance symptoms:

- **Migraine Relief**: A study published in the *Journal of Headache and Pain* found that DAO supplementation significantly reduced the duration of migraine attacks in individuals with a known deficiency (Maintz et al., 2011).
- **Digestive Health**: Research in the *Journal of Physiology and Pharmacology* demonstrated that DAO supplementation improved gastrointestinal symptoms, such as bloating and abdominal pain, in patients with histamine intolerance (Reese et al., 2014).
- **Histamine Degradation**: A study in *Clinical Gastroenterology and Hepatology* showed that oral DAO supplementation increased histamine degradation in the gut, reducing overall histamine levels (Manzotti et al., 2016).

## Conclusion

Diamine Oxidase (DAO) is a vital enzyme in the management of histamine levels, helping to prevent the symptoms associated with histamine intolerance. With a growing understanding of its role and the development of DAO supplements, individuals with histamine intolerance can find relief through targeted supplementation. As research continues, the potential applications and benefits of DAO will likely expand, offering hope for those affected by histamine-related conditions.

# Ginger

**Ginger**, a staple in traditional medicine, has been cherished for its potent medicinal properties and culinary versatility. This flowering plant, native to Southeast Asia, is renowned for its spicy, aromatic rhizome. Historically, it has been employed to treat a wide array of ailments, and modern science continues to uncover its diverse health benefits, especially its impact on allergies and histamine. Ginger's history dates back over 5,000 years, with its cultivation originating in the tropical rainforests of Southeast Asia. It has been utilized in various ancient medicinal systems, such as Ayurveda and Traditional Chinese Medicine (TCM), to treat digestive issues, pain, and inflammation. During the Roman Empire, ginger was highly prized and extensively traded, becoming a staple in European culinary and medicinal practices. Its popularity continued to grow during the Middle Ages, solidifying its status as a critical component of traditional medicine.

## Compounds and Ingredients

Ginger is rich in bioactive compounds, which contribute to its medicinal properties. The primary constituents include:

- **Gingerols**: These phenolic compounds are the main bioactive components in fresh ginger, responsible for its pungency and anti-inflammatory effects.
- **Shogaols**: Formed from gingerols during the drying process, shogaols are more potent and have stronger anti-inflammatory and antioxidant properties.
- **Paradols**: Found in lesser amounts, paradols also contribute to ginger's health benefits.
- **Zingerone**: A compound formed from gingerols upon heating, known for its anti-inflammatory and antioxidant properties.
- **Volatile Oils**: Such as zingiberene, contribute to ginger's aroma and have therapeutic effects.

## Mechanism of Action

The health benefits of ginger are attributed to its complex interplay of bioactive compounds. The primary mechanisms through which ginger exerts its effects include:

- **Anti-inflammatory Effects**: Gingerols and shogaols inhibit the production of pro-inflammatory cytokines and enzymes like COX-2, reducing inflammation and associated symptoms.
- **Antioxidant Properties**: Ginger neutralizes free radicals, reducing oxidative stress and protecting cells from damage.
- **Histamine Regulation**: By stabilizing mast cells, ginger reduces the release of histamine, alleviating symptoms of allergies and histamine intolerance.
- **Digestive Health**: Ginger stimulates digestive enzymes, enhances gastric motility, and reduces nausea and vomiting.

## Effects on Allergies and Histamine

Ginger's anti-inflammatory and mast cell-stabilizing properties make it a promising natural remedy for managing allergies and histamine intolerance. By inhibiting the release of histamine and other inflammatory mediators, ginger can help reduce symptoms such as itching, sneezing, nasal congestion, and gastrointestinal distress. Its antioxidative capacity further supports overall immune function and health.

## Recommended Doses

The recommended dose of ginger varies based on its form and intended use:

- **Fresh Ginger**: 1-2 grams per day, grated or sliced.
- **Ginger Powder**: 0.5-1 gram per day.
- **Ginger Tea**: 1-2 cups per day, made with fresh ginger slices or ginger powder.
- **Ginger Supplements**: 250-1,000 mg per day, depending on the concentration and formulation.

It's essential to start with lower doses to assess tolerance and consult with a healthcare provider before starting any new supplement regimen, especially for individuals with underlying health conditions or those taking other medications.

## Clinical Studies

Several clinical studies have highlighted the health benefits of ginger:

- **Nausea and Vomiting**: A study published in *Obstetrics & Gynecology* found that ginger was effective in reducing nausea and vomiting during pregnancy (Vutyavanich et al., 2001).
- **Inflammation and Pain**: Research in the *Journal of Pain* demonstrated that ginger supplementation reduced muscle pain and soreness following exercise-induced muscle injury (Black et al., 2010).

- **Digestive Health**: A study in the *World Journal of Gastroenterology* showed that ginger improved symptoms of indigestion and enhanced gastric motility (Hu et al., 2011).
- **Allergies and Asthma**: Research in the *American Journal of Physiology-Lung Cellular and Molecular Physiology* indicated that ginger extract could reduce airway inflammation and hyperresponsiveness in animal models of asthma (Akhani et al., 2014).

## Conclusion

Ginger is a versatile and potent natural remedy with a rich history of use and a wide array of health benefits. Its anti-inflammatory, antioxidant, and histamine-regulating properties make it an effective tool for managing allergies, histamine intolerance, and overall health. As research continues, ginger's potential applications and benefits will likely expand, solidifying its place as a cornerstone of natural medicine.

# Ginkgo Biloba

**Ginkgo biloba**, often referred to as a "living fossil," has captured the attention of researchers and herbalists for centuries. Ginkgo biloba, one of the oldest tree species on Earth, has a history dating back over 200 million years. It has been revered in traditional Chinese medicine for its therapeutic properties. Ancient texts describe its use for treating ailments such as asthma, bronchitis, and cognitive decline. Its survival through multiple mass extinctions and its continued use in modern herbal medicine underscore its significance and resilience.

## Compounds and Ingredients

The primary bioactive components of Ginkgo biloba are flavonoids and terpenoids:

- **Flavonoids:** These are powerful antioxidants that help combat oxidative stress by neutralizing free radicals. Key flavonoids in Ginkgo biloba include quercetin, kaempferol, and isorhamnetin.
- **Terpenoids:** These compounds, specifically ginkgolides and bilobalide, improve blood circulation by dilating blood vessels and reducing platelet aggregation. They also exhibit neuroprotective properties.

## Mechanism of Action

Ginkgo biloba operates through several mechanisms:

- **Antioxidant Action:** The flavonoids in Ginkgo biloba scavenge free radicals, reducing oxidative stress and preventing cellular damage.
- **Anti-inflammatory Effects:** By modulating inflammatory pathways, Ginkgo biloba can help reduce inflammation, which is beneficial for conditions like asthma and allergies.
- **Histamine Modulation:** Ginkgo biloba may stabilize mast cells, thereby reducing the release of histamine and alleviating allergy symptoms.
- **Neurotransmitter Regulation:** Ginkgo biloba enhances the uptake of neurotransmitters like dopamine and serotonin, potentially improving mood and cognitive function.

## Effects on Allergies and Histamine

Ginkgo biloba's potential anti-allergic properties are particularly noteworthy:

- **Reducing Histamine Release:** By stabilizing mast cells, Ginkgo biloba can prevent excessive histamine release, which is responsible for allergic reactions.
- **Anti-inflammatory Benefits:** Its anti-inflammatory properties help in reducing the severity of allergic responses.
- **Symptom Relief:** Some anecdotal evidence suggests Ginkgo biloba may alleviate symptoms such as nasal congestion, sneezing, and itchy eyes.

## Doses and Types for Consumption

Ginkgo biloba is available in various forms, including:

- **Standardized Extracts:** Typically standardized to contain 24% flavonoid glycosides and 6% terpenoids. The recommended dose ranges from 120 to 240 mg per day, divided into two or three doses.
- **Capsules and Tablets:** These are convenient for daily use.
- **Teas:** Less concentrated but can be a soothing way to consume Ginkgo biloba.
- **Liquid Extracts:** Allow for precise dosing but may have a bitter taste.

## Clinical Studies

Numerous clinical studies have investigated the effects of Ginkgo biloba, with varying results:

- **Cognitive Function:** Some studies suggest modest improvements in memory and cognitive performance, particularly in older adults with mild cognitive impairment or Alzheimer's disease.
- **Allergies and Asthma:** Preliminary studies indicate potential benefits in reducing allergy symptoms and improving asthma control.
- **Blood Circulation:** Ginkgo biloba has been shown to improve symptoms of peripheral artery disease and Raynaud's phenomenon.

### Conclusion

Ginkgo biloba is a remarkable herb with a range of potential health benefits. Its effects on allergies, histamine modulation, and cognitive function make it a subject of ongoing research. While promising, it is essential to consult healthcare professionals before incorporating Ginkgo biloba into your regimen to ensure safety and efficacy.

# Haridrakhand

**Haridrakhand**, also known as Haridra Khanda, is a classic Ayurvedic formulation renowned for its therapeutic properties, especially in treating allergies and inflammatory conditions. Haridrakhand has a deep-rooted history in Ayurveda, one of the world's oldest holistic healing systems. Dating back thousands of years, it is mentioned in ancient Ayurvedic texts such as the **Charaka Samhita** and **Ashtanga Hridayam**. Traditionally, it has been used to manage allergies, skin conditions, respiratory issues, and to enhance overall immunity.

## Compounds and Ingredients

The primary ingredient in Haridrakhand is **Haridra (Curcuma longa)**, commonly known as turmeric. Turmeric is renowned for its active compound **curcumin**, which has potent anti-inflammatory and antioxidant properties. Other significant ingredients in Haridrakhand include:

- **Trikatu (a blend of Piper longum, Piper nigrum, and Zingiber officinale)**
- **Sharkara** (sugar)
- **Ghrita** (clarified butter)
- **Ela (Elettaria cardamomum)**
- **Twak (Cinnamomum verum)**
- **Patra (Cinnamomum tamala)**

These ingredients work synergistically to enhance the formulation's therapeutic effects.

## Mechanism of Action

The efficacy of Haridrakhand can be attributed to its diverse pharmacological actions:

- **Anti-inflammatory Action**: Curcumin inhibits pro-inflammatory enzymes such as COX-2 and reduces the release of inflammatory cytokines. This helps in managing allergic reactions and reducing inflammation.
- **Antihistamine Properties**: Haridrakhand stabilizes mast cells, which are responsible for the release of histamine. By preventing histamine release, it

helps alleviate symptoms of allergic rhinitis and other histamine-related conditions.
- **Antioxidant Effects**: The formulation's antioxidant properties neutralize free radicals, reducing oxidative stress and promoting overall health.
- **Immunomodulation**: Haridrakhand enhances the body's immune response, helping to fight off infections and maintain immune homeostasis.

## Effects on Allergies and Histamine

Haridrakhand is particularly effective in managing allergies and histamine-related conditions. By inhibiting the release of histamine and other inflammatory mediators, it provides relief from common allergic symptoms such as itching, sneezing, and nasal congestion. The formulation's anti-inflammatory properties further enhance its effectiveness in treating allergic conditions.

## Recommended Doses

The recommended dosage of Haridrakhand varies based on age and individual health conditions:

- **Adults**: 5-10 grams, twice daily, mixed with warm milk or honey.
- **Children**: 1-2 grams, twice daily, mixed with warm milk or honey.

It is essential to consult with an Ayurvedic practitioner for personalized dosage recommendations.

## Types for Consumption

Haridrakhand is available in various forms, including:

- **Churna (Powder)**: The traditional form, usually mixed with warm milk or honey.
- **Tablets/Capsules**: Convenient for those who prefer not to taste the herbal blend.
- **Lehyam (Herbal Jam)**: A palatable form mixed with honey and ghee.

### Clinical Studies

Several clinical studies have highlighted the benefits of Haridrakhand:

- **Anti-Allergic Properties**: A study published in the Journal of Ayurveda and Integrative Medicine found that Haridrakhand significantly reduced symptoms of allergic rhinitis, such as nasal congestion and sneezing (Patil et al., 2014).

- **Anti-inflammatory Properties**: The herbs in Kashaya inhibit the production of pro-inflammatory cytokines and enzymes, reducing inflammation and associated symptoms.
- **Antioxidant Activity**: The presence of flavonoids and phenolic compounds helps neutralize free radicals, reducing oxidative stress.
- **Histamine Regulation**: Certain compounds in Kashaya stabilize mast cells, preventing the release of histamine and other inflammatory mediators, thereby alleviating allergic symptoms.
- **Digestive Health**: Ingredients like ginger and coriander improve digestion and enhance nutrient absorption, supporting overall health and immunity.
- **Immune Modulation**: Kashaya boosts the body's immune response, making it more resilient to infections and allergens.

## Effects on Allergies and Histamine

Kashaya is effective in managing allergies and histamine-related conditions due to its anti-inflammatory and antihistamine properties. By stabilizing mast cells and preventing histamine release, Kashaya helps reduce symptoms like itching, sneezing, and nasal congestion. Its immune-boosting and antioxidant effects further enhance its ability to manage allergic reactions and support respiratory health.

## Recommended Doses

The recommended dose of Kashaya can vary depending on the formulation and the individual's health condition:

- **General Dosage**: Typically, 1-2 tablespoons of Kashaya powder mixed with 200 ml of boiling water, consumed once or twice daily.
- **For Specific Conditions**: The dosage may be adjusted based on the severity of the condition and the specific ingredients used. It is advisable to consult an Ayurvedic practitioner for personalized dosage recommendations.

## Types for Consumption

Kashaya can be consumed in various forms to suit different preferences:

- **Decoction (Kwath)**: The traditional method involves boiling the herbs in water to extract their medicinal properties.
- **Powder (Churna)**: The dried herbs are ground into a fine powder, which can be mixed with water or other liquids.
- **Tablets/Capsules**: Standardized extracts are available in pill form for convenient dosing.

## Clinical Studies

Several clinical studies have explored the health benefits of Kashaya:

- **Anti-Allergic Effects**: A study published in the Journal of Ethnopharmacology found that Kashaya formulations significantly reduced allergic symptoms by inhibiting histamine release and reducing inflammation (Sharma et al., 2013).
- **Anti-Inflammatory Properties**: Research in the International Journal of Ayurveda Research demonstrated that Kashaya formulations have potent anti-inflammatory effects, reducing markers of inflammation in patients with chronic inflammatory conditions (Patil et al., 2016).
- **Digestive Health**: A clinical trial in the Journal of Ayurveda and Integrative Medicine showed that Kashaya improves digestive health and supports the balance of beneficial gut bacteria, enhancing overall immune function (Kumar et al., 2017).

## Conclusion

Kashaya is a versatile Ayurvedic remedy with a rich history and a wide range of therapeutic benefits. Its bioactive compounds, anti-inflammatory, antioxidant, and antihistamine properties make it an effective natural treatment for managing allergies and supporting overall health. However, it is essential to use Kashaya under the guidance of a qualified Ayurvedic practitioner to ensure safety and efficacy.

# Lactobacillus Plantarum

**Lactobacillus plantarum** is a versatile and widely studied probiotic bacterium known for its numerous health benefits. Lactobacillus plantarum is commonly found in fermented foods such as sauerkraut, kimchi, pickles, and sourdough bread. It has been utilized for centuries in traditional fermentation practices to enhance food preservation and flavor. The probiotic properties of Lactobacillus plantarum were later discovered, leading to its use in promoting gut health and overall well-being.

## Compounds and Ingredients

- **Lactic Acid:** Produced during fermentation, lactic acid helps maintain an acidic environment in the gut, inhibiting the growth of harmful bacteria.
- **Bacteriocins:** These antimicrobial peptides target and kill pathogenic bacteria, contributing to a balanced gut microbiome.
- **Exopolysaccharides:** These complex sugars have immunomodulatory and anti-inflammatory properties, which may help in managing allergies and inflammatory conditions.

## Mechanism of Action

- **Modulation of Gut Microbiota:** By promoting the growth of beneficial bacteria and inhibiting pathogens, Lactobacillus plantarum helps maintain a healthy and balanced gut microbiome.
- **Immune System Regulation:** Lactobacillus plantarum interacts with the immune system, enhancing its ability to respond to infections and reducing excessive inflammatory responses.
- **Histamine Degradation:** This probiotic can break down histamine, potentially reducing histamine-related symptoms such as allergic reactions, headaches, and digestive issues.
- **Anti-inflammatory Effects:** Lactobacillus plantarum produces compounds that can reduce inflammation, which may be beneficial for conditions like irritable bowel syndrome (IBS) and allergies.

## Effects on Allergies and Histamine

- **Histamine Degradation:** By breaking down histamine, Lactobacillus plantarum can alleviate symptoms related to histamine intolerance, such as rashes, hives, and gastrointestinal discomfort.
- **Immune Modulation:** Its ability to regulate the immune system helps reduce the severity of allergic responses.
- **Symptom Relief:** Clinical studies and anecdotal evidence suggest that Lactobacillus plantarum may help reduce symptoms of allergic rhinitis, asthma, and eczema.

## Doses and Types for Consumption

- **Probiotic Supplements:** Available in capsules, tablets, and powders. The recommended dose typically ranges from 1 billion to 10 billion CFUs (colony-forming units) per day, depending on the specific product and health condition.
- **Fermented Foods:** Consuming naturally fermented foods like sauerkraut, kimchi, and yogurt can provide a natural source of Lactobacillus plantarum.
- **Functional Foods and Beverages:** Some foods and beverages are fortified with Lactobacillus plantarum to enhance their probiotic content.

# Clinical Studies

Numerous clinical studies have explored the effects of Lactobacillus plantarum:

- **Allergies:** Studies suggest that Lactobacillus plantarum may help reduce symptoms of allergic rhinitis, asthma, and eczema by modulating the immune response and degrading histamine.
- **Gut Health:** Research indicates that Lactobacillus plantarum can improve symptoms of IBS, reduce gut inflammation, and promote a balanced gut microbiome.
- **Overall Health:** Additional studies suggest potential benefits in reducing cholesterol levels, supporting weight management, and enhancing immune function.

# Conclusion

Lactobacillus plantarum is a versatile probiotic with a range of potential health benefits. Its effects on allergies, histamine degradation, and gut health make it a subject of ongoing research. While promising, it is essential to consult healthcare professionals before incorporating Lactobacillus plantarum into your regimen to ensure safety and efficacy.

# Lactobacillus Rhamnosus

**Lactobacillus rhamnosus** is a well-researched probiotic strain known for its numerous health benefits. Lactobacillus rhamnosus has been a staple in fermented foods for centuries, contributing to the preservation and enhancement of food flavors. This probiotic strain was later isolated and studied for its health benefits, particularly in promoting gut health and boosting the immune system.

## Compounds and Ingredients

Lactobacillus rhamnosus produces several beneficial compounds:

- **Lactic Acid:** Helps maintain an acidic environment in the gut, inhibiting the growth of harmful bacteria.
- **Bacteriocins:** These antimicrobial peptides target and kill pathogenic bacteria, contributing to a balanced gut microbiome.
- **Exopolysaccharides:** Complex sugars that have immunomodulatory and anti-inflammatory properties, which may help in managing allergies and inflammatory conditions.

## Mechanism of Action

Lactobacillus rhamnosus exerts its beneficial effects through multiple mechanisms:

- **Modulation of Gut Microbiota:** Promotes the growth of beneficial bacteria and inhibits pathogens, helping maintain a healthy and balanced gut microbiome.
- **Immune System Regulation:** Interacts with the immune system, enhancing its ability to respond to infections and reducing excessive inflammatory responses.
- **Histamine Degradation:** This probiotic can break down histamine, potentially reducing histamine-related symptoms such as allergic reactions, headaches, and digestive issues.
- **Anti-inflammatory Effects:** Produces compounds that can reduce inflammation, which may be beneficial for conditions like irritable bowel syndrome (IBS) and allergies.

## Effects on Allergies and Histamine

- **Histamine Degradation:** By breaking down histamine, Lactobacillus rhamnosus can alleviate symptoms related to histamine intolerance, such as rashes, hives, and gastrointestinal discomfort.
- **Immune Modulation:** Its ability to regulate the immune system helps reduce the severity of allergic responses.
- **Symptom Relief:** Clinical studies and anecdotal evidence suggest that Lactobacillus rhamnosus may help reduce symptoms of allergic rhinitis, asthma, and eczema.

## Doses and Types for Consumption

- **Probiotic Supplements:** Available in capsules, tablets, and powders. The recommended dose typically ranges from 1 billion to 10 billion CFUs (colony-forming units) per day, depending on the specific product and health condition.
- **Fermented Foods:** Consuming naturally fermented foods like yogurt, kefir, and cheese can provide a natural source of Lactobacillus rhamnosus.
- **Functional Foods and Beverages:** Some foods and beverages are fortified with Lactobacillus rhamnosus to enhance their probiotic content.

## Clinical Studies

- **Allergies:** Studies suggest that Lactobacillus rhamnosus may help reduce symptoms of allergic rhinitis, asthma, and eczema by modulating the immune response and degrading histamine.
- **Gut Health:** Research indicates that Lactobacillus rhamnosus can improve symptoms of IBS, reduce gut inflammation, and promote a balanced gut microbiome.
- **Overall Health:** Additional studies suggest potential benefits in reducing cholesterol levels, supporting weight management, and enhancing immune function.

## Conclusion

Lactobacillus rhamnosus is a versatile probiotic with a range of potential health benefits. Its effects on allergies, histamine degradation, and gut health make it a subject of ongoing research. While promising, it is essential to consult healthcare professionals before incorporating Lactobacillus rhamnosus into your regimen to ensure safety and efficacy.

# Liquorice Root

**Liquorice root**, derived from the plant Glycyrrhiza glabra, has been used for centuries across various cultures for its medicinal properties. This herb is celebrated for its sweet flavor and myriad health benefits, particularly its effects on allergies, histamine regulation, and overall immune function. Liquorice root has a rich history of use in traditional medicine systems around the world, dating back thousands of years. In ancient Egypt, it was used to make a sweet drink favored by pharaohs. In traditional Chinese medicine (TCM), liquorice root is known as **Gan Cao** and is often used as a harmonizing agent in herbal formulas. It is also a staple in Ayurveda, where it is referred to as Yashtimadhu and used to treat respiratory issues, digestive problems, and skin conditions.

## Compounds and Ingredients

Liquorice root contains over 300 compounds, with the most prominent being:

- **Glycyrrhizin**: A saponin responsible for the sweet taste and many of the root's medicinal properties.
- **Flavonoids**: Including liquiritin, isoliquiritin, and glabridin, which possess antioxidant and anti-inflammatory properties.
- **Coumarins**: Such as herniarin and umbelliferone, which contribute to its therapeutic effects.
- **Polysaccharides**: Which support immune function and promote overall health.

## Mechanism of Action

The primary mechanisms through which liquorice root exerts its effects include:

- **Anti-inflammatory Properties**: Glycyrrhizin inhibits enzymes involved in inflammation, such as cyclooxygenase (COX) and lipoxygenase (LOX), reducing the production of pro-inflammatory cytokines.
- **Histamine Regulation**: Liquorice root's compounds stabilize mast cells, preventing the release of histamine, which is crucial in managing allergic reactions.
- **Immune Modulation**: It enhances the production of interferons and natural killer cells, boosting the body's defense mechanisms.

- **Cortisol Mimicry**: Glycyrrhizin inhibits the enzyme 11β-hydroxysteroid dehydrogenase, leading to increased levels of cortisol, which has anti-inflammatory and immune-modulating effects.

## Effects on Allergies and Histamine

Liquorice root is particularly effective in managing allergies and histamine-related conditions. By stabilizing mast cells and preventing histamine release, it alleviates symptoms such as itching, sneezing, and nasal congestion. Its anti-inflammatory properties further reduce the severity of allergic reactions, making it a valuable natural remedy for conditions like allergic rhinitis, asthma, and eczema.

## Recommended Doses

The recommended dose of liquorice root varies depending on the form and purpose of use:

- **Powder**: 1-3 grams per day, typically mixed with warm water or milk.
- **Capsules/Tablets**: 250-500 mg of standardized extract, taken once or twice daily.
- **Tincture**: 1-2 ml, taken up to three times daily.

It is important to consult with a healthcare provider for personalized dosage recommendations, especially when using high doses or for prolonged periods, as excessive consumption can lead to side effects like hypertension and electrolyte imbalances.

## Types for Consumption

Liquorice root can be consumed in various forms to suit different preferences and needs:

- **Tea**: Made by steeping dried liquorice root in hot water.
- **Capsules/Tablets**: Convenient for those who prefer a precise dosage without the taste.
- **Tinctures**: Alcohol-based extracts that provide a concentrated form of the root's active compounds.
- **Topical Applications**: Creams and ointments containing liquorice root extract are used to treat skin conditions such as eczema and psoriasis.

## Clinical Studies

Several clinical studies have explored the health benefits of liquorice root:

- **Anti-Allergic Effects**: A study published in Phytotherapy Research found that liquorice root extract significantly reduced allergic symptoms in patients with allergic rhinitis by stabilizing mast cells and reducing histamine release (Shin et al., 2014).
- **Anti-Inflammatory Properties**: Research in the Journal of Ethnopharmacology demonstrated that glycyrrhizin reduces inflammation by inhibiting pro-inflammatory enzymes and cytokines (Asl & Hosseinzadeh, 2008).
- **Immune Modulation**: A study in the Journal of Immunology Research showed that liquorice root enhances the body's immune response by increasing the production of interferons and natural killer cells (Fiore et al., 2008).

## Conclusion

Liquorice root is a versatile herb with a long history of use in traditional medicine. Its bioactive compounds, particularly glycyrrhizin, provide a range of therapeutic benefits, including anti-inflammatory, anti-allergic, and immune-modulating effects. However, it is essential to use liquorice root responsibly and under the guidance of a healthcare provider to avoid potential side effects and ensure safe and effective use.

# Luteolin

**Luteolin** is a naturally occurring flavonoid found in various plants, known for its extensive health benefits. Luteolin has been part of human diet and medicine for centuries. Found in a wide variety of plants, luteolin has been used in traditional remedies across cultures. Ancient civilizations utilized plants rich in luteolin for their anti-inflammatory, antimicrobial, and antioxidant properties. The isolation of luteolin in the 19th century marked the beginning of modern scientific investigations into its potential health benefits.

## Compounds and Ingredients

Luteolin is a flavonoid, specifically a flavone, characterized by a structure of two benzene rings connected by a three-carbon bridge, forming a pyran ring. Its molecular formula is $C_{15}H_{10}O_6$. It is commonly found in plants such as celery, parsley, thyme, and chamomile. Luteolin can exist in both free and glycosylated forms, the latter being more common in nature and converted to free luteolin during digestion.

## Mechanism of Action

Luteolin exerts its biological effects through multiple pathways:

- **Antioxidant Activity:** Luteolin scavenges free radicals, reduces oxidative stress, and prevents cellular damage.
- **Anti-inflammatory Effects:** It inhibits the production of pro-inflammatory cytokines and enzymes, thereby reducing inflammation.
- **Mast Cell Stabilization:** Luteolin stabilizes mast cells, which release histamine and other mediators during allergic reactions.
- **Histamine Modulation:** By inhibiting the release of histamine, luteolin can reduce symptoms of allergies and histamine intolerance.
- **Enzyme Inhibition:** It inhibits enzymes like phosphodiesterase and lipoxygenase, which play roles in inflammation and allergic responses.

## Effects on Allergies and Histamine

Luteolin has shown significant potential in managing allergies and histamine-related conditions:

- **Allergic Reactions:** Luteolin's ability to stabilize mast cells and inhibit histamine release makes it effective in reducing symptoms of allergies, such as itching, swelling, and redness.
- **Anti-inflammatory Benefits:** By reducing the production of inflammatory cytokines, luteolin can help manage chronic inflammatory conditions, including asthma and dermatitis.
- **Histamine Intolerance:** Luteolin's role in degrading histamine can alleviate symptoms like headaches, digestive issues, and skin reactions associated with histamine intolerance.

## Recommended Doses

The optimal dosage of luteolin can vary depending on the intended use and individual factors. Common supplemental doses range from **100 mg to 500 mg per day**. It is crucial to consult a healthcare provider before starting any new supplement to ensure safety and efficacy.

## Types for Consumption

Luteolin can be consumed through dietary sources and supplements:

- **Dietary Sources:** Foods rich in luteolin include celery, parsley, thyme, chamomile tea, and green peppers.
- **Supplements:** Luteolin supplements are available in capsules, tablets, and powders. These supplements often provide a more concentrated dose of luteolin than dietary sources.
- **Functional Foods:** Some foods and beverages are fortified with luteolin to enhance their health benefits.

## Clinical Studies

Several clinical studies have investigated the health benefits of luteolin:

- **Inflammation and Allergies:** Research has shown luteolin's effectiveness in reducing inflammatory markers and improving symptoms of allergic conditions.
- **Neuroprotection:** Studies suggest that luteolin may have neuroprotective effects, potentially benefiting conditions like Alzheimer's disease and cognitive decline.
- **Cancer:** Preliminary studies indicate that luteolin may inhibit the growth of certain cancer cells and enhance the efficacy of chemotherapy.

## Conclusion

Luteolin is a promising natural compound with a broad spectrum of health benefits. Its antioxidant, anti-inflammatory, and antihistamine properties make it a valuable addition to the diet for managing allergies and other inflammatory conditions. However, further research is needed to fully understand its mechanisms and optimize its use in clinical settings.

# Methylsulfonylmethane (MSM)

**Methylsulfonylmethane (MSM)** is an organic sulfur compound found naturally in various foods and present in small amounts in the human body. Known for its anti-inflammatory and antioxidant properties, MSM has gained popularity as a supplement for managing pain, allergies, and other health conditions. MSM was first discovered during research on dimethyl sulfoxide (DMSO) in the 1950s. Researchers noted that MSM, a metabolite of DMSO, also exhibited significant therapeutic properties. Since then, MSM has been widely studied for its potential health benefits and is now commonly used as a dietary supplement.

## Compounds

MSM is a sulfur-containing compound with the chemical formula $(CH_3)_2SO_2$. It is an important source of sulfur, a mineral that plays a crucial role in various bodily functions, including the formation of connective tissue, enzyme function, and detoxification processes. The primary bioactive ingredient in MSM is sulfur, which is essential for maintaining healthy joints, skin, hair, and nails.

## Mechanism of Action

MSM exerts its effects through several mechanisms:

- **Anti-inflammatory Activity:** MSM inhibits the production of pro-inflammatory cytokines, reducing inflammation and associated pain.
- **Antioxidant Properties:** MSM enhances the production of glutathione, a potent antioxidant that protects cells from oxidative damage.
- **Histamine Modulation:** MSM may help regulate histamine levels in the body, reducing allergic reactions and histamine intolerance symptoms.
- **Joint and Connective Tissue Support:** MSM contributes to the formation of collagen and keratin, essential for maintaining healthy joints, skin, hair, and nails.

## Effects on Allergies and Histamine

MSM has shown promise in alleviating symptoms of allergies and histamine intolerance. By modulating the body's histamine response and reducing inflammation, MSM can help alleviate common allergic symptoms such as sneezing, nasal congestion, and itching. Clinical studies have demonstrated that MSM supplementation can significantly reduce symptoms of seasonal allergic rhinitis (SAR).

## Recommended Doses

The optimal dosage of MSM can vary depending on the condition being treated and individual factors. Common dosages range from **1,000 mg to 6,000 mg per day**, divided into two or three doses. It is recommended to start with a lower dose and gradually increase it to minimize potential side effects. Consulting a healthcare provider before starting MSM supplementation is essential for determining the appropriate dosage.

## Types for Consumption

MSM is available in various forms, including:

- **Capsules and Tablets:** Convenient for oral consumption and come in various dosages.
- **Powders:** Can be mixed with water or other beverages for easy consumption.
- **Creams and Gels:** Applied topically to target specific areas of pain or inflammation.
- **Natural Sources:** Found in small amounts in foods like fruits, vegetables, grains, and animal products.

## Clinical Studies

Numerous clinical studies have investigated the effects of MSM on various health conditions:

- **Allergies:** Studies have shown that MSM can reduce symptoms of seasonal allergic rhinitis, including nasal congestion, sneezing, and coughing.
- **Osteoarthritis:** Research indicates that MSM can significantly reduce pain and improve joint function in individuals with osteoarthritis.
- **Exercise Recovery:** MSM has been found to reduce muscle soreness and improve recovery time in athletes following intense exercise.
- **Inflammation and Pain:** Studies suggest that MSM can effectively reduce inflammation and pain in conditions like rheumatoid arthritis and inflammatory bowel disease.

## Conclusion

MSM is a versatile and promising supplement with a range of potential health benefits, particularly in reducing inflammation and alleviating pain. Its effects on allergies and histamine make it a valuable option for individuals with allergic conditions and histamine intolerance. While more research is needed to fully understand its mechanisms and establish optimal dosages, MSM remains a popular choice for those seeking natural remedies for inflammation and pain.

# N-Acetyl-L-Cysteine (NAC)

**N-Acetyl-L-Cysteine (NAC)** is a powerful antioxidant and supplement that has gained attention for its potential health benefits. N-Acetyl-L-Cysteine has a long history of use in medical practice. It was first introduced in the 1960s as a mucolytic agent to treat chronic respiratory conditions by breaking down mucus. Over the years, its applications have expanded to include treatment for acetaminophen overdose, mental health disorders, and as an antioxidant supplement.

## Compounds and Ingredients

NAC is a derivative of the amino acid L-cysteine and serves as a precursor to glutathione, one of the body's most important antioxidants. The primary ingredient in NAC supplements is N-Acetyl-L-Cysteine itself, often combined with other supportive nutrients to enhance its effects.

## Mechanism of Action

- **Antioxidant Production:** By replenishing intracellular glutathione levels, NAC helps reduce oxidative stress and protect cells from damage.
- **Detoxification:** NAC aids in detoxification processes in the liver, particularly in neutralizing acetaminophen toxicity.
- **Mucolytic Activity:** It breaks disulfide bonds in mucus, reducing its viscosity and aiding in clearance from the respiratory tract.
- **Immune System Modulation:** NAC modulates the immune response, potentially reducing inflammation and histamine release.

## Effects on Allergies and Histamine

NAC has shown promise in managing allergies and histamine-related conditions:

- **Histamine Degradation:** NAC may help regulate histamine levels, thereby alleviating symptoms associated with histamine intolerance, such as headaches, hives, and gastrointestinal issues.
- **Anti-inflammatory Properties:** By reducing oxidative stress and inflammation, NAC can potentially reduce the severity of allergic responses and asthma symptoms.
- **Immune System Support:** NAC's ability to modulate immune function may contribute to a balanced response to allergens.

# Recommended Doses

The optimal dosage of NAC can vary depending on the condition being treated. Common doses for general antioxidant support range from 600 mg to 1200 mg per day. For specific conditions like respiratory issues or acetaminophen overdose, higher doses may be recommended under medical supervision.

# Types for Consumption

- **Oral Supplements:** Capsules and tablets are the most common forms, providing a convenient way to take NAC.
- **Powders:** NAC in powder form can be mixed with water or other beverages.
- **Inhalation:** For respiratory conditions, NAC can be administered as an inhalant to break down mucus.
- **Intravenous:** In medical settings, NAC is administered intravenously for acute conditions like acetaminophen overdose.

# Clinical Studies

- **Respiratory Health:** Studies have shown that NAC can help improve symptoms of chronic bronchitis and COPD by reducing mucus viscosity and improving clearance.
- **Mental Health:** Research indicates that NAC may benefit conditions like depression, anxiety, and obsessive-compulsive disorder by modulating glutamate levels and reducing oxidative stress.
- **Liver Health:** NAC is well-established as an effective treatment for acetaminophen toxicity, helping to prevent liver damage by replenishing glutathione levels.

# Conclusion

N-Acetyl-L-Cysteine is a versatile and powerful compound with a wide range of potential health benefits. Its effects on allergies, histamine regulation, and overall antioxidant support make it a valuable addition to many health regimens. As with any supplement, it is essential to consult healthcare professionals before incorporating NAC to ensure safe and effective use.

# Omega-3 Fatty Acids

**Omega-3 fatty acids** are essential polyunsaturated fats that play a critical role in human health. These fats are not synthesized by the body and must be obtained through diet or supplementation. The recognition of Omega-3 fatty acids' health benefits can be traced back to the 1970s when researchers observed low rates of cardiovascular diseases among the Inuit people of Greenland, whose diet was rich in fatty fish. Since then, Omega-3s have been widely studied and incorporated into dietary guidelines across the globe. Historically, fish oil has been used for its medicinal properties, with early records suggesting its use in treating joint pain and skin conditions.

## Compounds and Ingredients

Omega-3 fatty acids consist of three main types:

- **Alpha-linolenic acid (ALA):** Found in plant oils, such as flaxseed, soybean, and chia seeds. ALA is a short-chain Omega-3 that can be partially converted into EPA and DHA in the body.
- **Eicosapentaenoic acid (EPA):** Found in marine sources like fish oil and algae. EPA plays a vital role in reducing inflammation and improving cardiovascular health.
- **Docosahexaenoic acid (DHA):** Also found in marine sources, DHA is essential for brain health, vision, and neural development.

## Mechanism of Action

Omega-3 fatty acids exert their effects through several biological mechanisms:

- **Anti-inflammatory Properties:** Omega-3s inhibit the production of pro-inflammatory cytokines and eicosanoids derived from arachidonic acid. They promote the production of anti-inflammatory eicosanoids, reducing inflammation.
- **Cell Membrane Fluidity:** Incorporation of EPA and DHA into cell membranes enhances membrane fluidity, improving cell signaling and function.
- **Gene Expression Modulation:** Omega-3s influence the expression of genes involved in inflammation, lipid metabolism, and cellular function.

- **Histamine Regulation:** Omega-3 fatty acids can reduce histamine release from mast cells, potentially alleviating symptoms of allergies and histamine intolerance.

## Effects on Allergies and Histamine

Omega-3 fatty acids have shown promise in managing allergies and histamine-related conditions:

- **Anti-inflammatory Benefits:** By reducing the production of pro-inflammatory cytokines, Omega-3s can help manage chronic inflammatory conditions, including asthma and eczema.
- **Histamine Modulation:** Omega-3s can lower histamine levels, alleviating symptoms of histamine intolerance such as headaches, hives, and digestive discomfort.
- **Immune Support:** Omega-3s contribute to a balanced immune response, potentially reducing the severity of allergic reactions.

## Recommended Doses

The optimal dosage of Omega-3 fatty acids varies depending on individual health needs. The American Heart Association recommends consuming at least two servings of fatty fish per week, equivalent to approximately 500 mg of EPA and DHA per day. For individuals with specific health conditions, higher doses may be prescribed by healthcare professionals.

## Types for Consumption

Omega-3 fatty acids can be consumed through various sources:

- **Dietary Sources:** Fatty fish (salmon, mackerel, sardines), flaxseed, chia seeds, walnuts, and algae.
- **Supplements:** Fish oil capsules, krill oil, algae-based supplements, and fortified foods.
- **Functional Foods:** Some foods and beverages are enriched with Omega-3s to enhance their nutritional value.

## Clinical Studies

Numerous clinical studies have investigated the health benefits of Omega-3 fatty acids:

- **Cardiovascular Health:** Research has shown that Omega-3 supplementation can reduce the risk of heart attacks, strokes, and other

cardiovascular diseases by improving lipid profiles and reducing inflammation.
- **Cognitive Function:** Studies suggest that DHA is crucial for brain health and may help improve cognitive function and reduce the risk of neurodegenerative diseases.
- **Inflammatory Conditions:** Omega-3s have been found to alleviate symptoms of rheumatoid arthritis, inflammatory bowel disease, and asthma.
- **Allergies and Histamine Intolerance:** Clinical trials indicate that Omega-3 supplementation can reduce the severity of allergic rhinitis and improve symptoms of histamine intolerance.

## Conclusion

Omega-3 fatty acids are essential nutrients with a wide range of health benefits. Their anti-inflammatory properties, histamine regulation, and overall support for cardiovascular and cognitive health make them a valuable addition to any diet. While more research is needed to fully understand their mechanisms and optimize their use, the existing evidence supports the significant role of Omega-3s in promoting health and preventing disease.

# Palmitoylethanolamide (PEA)

**Palmitoylethanolamide (PEA)** is a naturally occurring lipid mediator that has garnered significant attention for its potential therapeutic effects, particularly in managing pain, inflammation, allergies, and histamine-related conditions. The discovery of PEA dates back to the 1950s when it was first identified in egg yolk. It was later found in various foods such as peanuts, soybeans, and egg yolk. Early studies recognized its anti-inflammatory properties, and over time, PEA has been investigated for its potential in treating chronic pain, neuroinflammation, and immune modulation. Its usage has expanded significantly, particularly in European countries, where it is commonly used as a supplement for various inflammatory and pain conditions.

## Compounds and Ingredients

PEA is a fatty acid amide and part of the N-acylethanolamine family. It is an endogenous compound, meaning it is produced naturally in the body. PEA is composed of palmitic acid and ethanolamine. It is structurally similar to anandamide, an endocannabinoid, but does not directly interact with cannabinoid receptors. PEA is often formulated with other ingredients to enhance its bioavailability and efficacy, such as alpha-lipoic acid, quercetin, and luteolin.

## Mechanism of Action

PEA exerts its therapeutic effects through multiple mechanisms:

- **Activation of PPAR-α:** PEA activates peroxisome proliferator-activated receptor-alpha (PPAR-α), which modulates the expression of genes involved in inflammation and pain. Activation of PPAR-α leads to anti-inflammatory and analgesic effects.
- **Mast Cell Stabilization:** PEA downregulates mast cell degranulation, thereby reducing the release of histamine and other pro-inflammatory mediators, which can help mitigate allergic reactions.
- **Endocannabinoid System Modulation:** Although PEA does not bind directly to cannabinoid receptors, it enhances the levels of anandamide by inhibiting its degradation, indirectly exerting anti-inflammatory and neuroprotective effects.

- **Interaction with TRPV1 Receptors:** PEA interacts with transient receptor potential vanilloid 1 (TRPV1) receptors, contributing to its analgesic properties.
- **Neuroprotection:** PEA exerts neuroprotective effects by reducing neuroinflammation and oxidative stress, which can be beneficial in conditions like multiple sclerosis and Alzheimer's disease.

## Effects on Allergies and Histamine

PEA has shown promise in managing allergies and histamine-related conditions through the following mechanisms:

- **Histamine Modulation:** By stabilizing mast cells, PEA reduces the release of histamine, alleviating symptoms such as itching, swelling, and redness.
- **Anti-inflammatory Properties:** PEA's ability to activate PPAR-α and reduce pro-inflammatory cytokines helps manage chronic inflammatory conditions, including allergic rhinitis, asthma, and atopic dermatitis.
- **Immune Modulation:** PEA supports a balanced immune response, potentially reducing the severity of allergic reactions and enhancing overall immune function.

## Recommended Doses

The optimal dosage of PEA can vary depending on individual health needs and conditions. Typical doses range **from 300 mg to 1,200 mg per day**, divided into two or three doses. For chronic pain and severe inflammation, higher doses may be necessary, under medical supervision.

## Types for Consumption

PEA is available in various forms, including:

- **Oral Supplements:** Capsules and tablets are the most common forms, providing a convenient way to take PEA.
- **Topical Formulations:** Creams and lotions can be applied directly to the skin for localized relief of pain and inflammation.
- **Micronized and Ultramicronized Forms:** These forms enhance the bioavailability of PEA, making it more effective at lower doses.

## Clinical Studies

Numerous clinical studies have explored the health benefits of PEA:

- **Pain Management:** A randomized controlled trial demonstrated that PEA supplementation significantly reduced pain intensity in patients with chronic pain conditions such as osteoarthritis and sciatic pain.
- **Allergic Rhinitis:** A double-blind, placebo-controlled study found that PEA reduced symptoms of allergic rhinitis, including nasal congestion and itching, by modulating the immune response and reducing histamine release.
- **Neuroinflammation:** Research indicates that PEA may have neuroprotective effects, reducing neuroinflammation and improving cognitive function in conditions like multiple sclerosis and Alzheimer's disease.
- **Atopic Dermatitis:** Clinical trials have shown that PEA can reduce the severity of atopic dermatitis by decreasing skin inflammation and itching.

## Conclusion

Palmitoylethanolamide is a promising lipid mediator with a wide range of potential therapeutic benefits. Its effects on allergies, histamine regulation, pain management, and neuroprotection make it a valuable addition to the treatment of various inflammatory and allergic conditions. As with any supplement, it is essential to consult healthcare professionals before incorporating PEA to ensure safe and effective use.

# Probiotics

**Probiotics**, often referred to as "good bacteria," are live microorganisms that confer health benefits to the host when consumed in adequate amounts. They are found in fermented foods, dietary supplements, and even in certain functional foods. The concept of probiotics dates back to the early 20th century when Russian scientist Elie Metchnikoff observed the health benefits of fermented milk products consumed by Bulgarian villagers. Metchnikoff's pioneering work at the Pasteur Institute in Paris laid the groundwork for modern probiotic research. He proposed that consuming beneficial bacteria could enhance gut health and increase longevity. Since then, probiotics have become an integral part of health and wellness, with ongoing research exploring their vast potential.

## Compounds and Ingredients

Probiotics comprise various strains of beneficial bacteria and yeasts. The most common and well-researched probiotic strains include:

- **Lactobacillus:** Species such as Lactobacillus acidophilus, Lactobacillus rhamnosus, and Lactobacillus plantarum are known for their gut health benefits.
- **Bifidobacterium:** Species like Bifidobacterium bifidum and Bifidobacterium longum play crucial roles in maintaining a healthy gut microbiota.
- **Saccharomyces boulardii:** A beneficial yeast that helps combat gastrointestinal disorders. These strains are typically found in fermented foods and dietary supplements, working synergistically to promote overall well-being.

## Mechanisms of Action

Probiotics exert their beneficial effects through several mechanisms:

- **Gut Microbiota Modulation:** Probiotics enhance the balance of gut microbiota, promoting the growth of beneficial bacteria and inhibiting harmful pathogens. This balance is crucial for maintaining gut health and immune function.
- **Barrier Function Enhancement:** Probiotics strengthen the gut barrier, preventing the translocation of harmful bacteria and toxins into the bloodstream, thereby reducing inflammation.

- **Immune System Modulation:** Probiotics interact with the gut-associated lymphoid tissue (GALT) to modulate immune responses. They enhance the production of anti-inflammatory cytokines and suppress pro-inflammatory pathways.
- **Histamine Degradation:** Certain probiotic strains can degrade histamine, helping to alleviate symptoms of histamine intolerance, such as headaches, skin rashes, and gastrointestinal discomfort.

## Effects on Allergies

Probiotics have shown significant promise in managing allergies by modulating the immune system and reducing inflammation. Research has demonstrated that probiotics can alleviate symptoms of allergic rhinitis, atopic dermatitis, and food allergies. For instance, a systematic review and meta-analysis published in the *American Journal of Clinical Nutrition* found that probiotic supplementation significantly improved symptoms of allergic rhinitis, including nasal congestion and itching.

## Recommended Doses

The appropriate dose of probiotics varies depending on the specific strain and the health condition being addressed. Generally, doses range from 1 billion to 100 billion colony-forming units (CFUs) per day. It is essential to follow the manufacturer's recommendations and consult with a healthcare professional to determine the optimal dose for your needs.

## Types for Consumption

Probiotics can be consumed through various forms, including:

- **Fermented Foods:** Yogurt, kefir, sauerkraut, kimchi, miso, and tempeh are rich sources of probiotics.
- **Dietary Supplements:** Probiotic supplements are available in capsules, tablets, powders, and liquid forms. These supplements often contain specific strains targeted for particular health benefits.
- **Functional Foods:** Some foods and beverages are fortified with probiotics, such as probiotic-enriched juices and snack bars.

## Clinical Studies

Numerous clinical studies have investigated the health benefits of probiotics:

- **Allergic Rhinitis:** A randomized controlled trial published in *Clinical & Experimental Allergy* demonstrated that Lactobacillus paracasei

supplementation reduced symptoms and improved quality of life in patients with allergic rhinitis.
- **Atopic Dermatitis:** A study in *The Journal of Allergy and Clinical Immunology* found that probiotics, particularly Lactobacillus rhamnosus, reduced the severity of atopic dermatitis in children.
- **Histamine Intolerance:** Research in *Clinical and Translational Allergy* highlighted that certain probiotic strains can degrade histamine, thereby alleviating symptoms associated with histamine intolerance.
- **Gut Health:** A meta-analysis in *PLOS ONE* confirmed that probiotics improve symptoms of irritable bowel syndrome (IBS) by modulating gut microbiota and reducing inflammation.

## Conclusion

Probiotics offer a natural and effective way to support gut health and overall well-being. Their ability to modulate the immune system, reduce histamine levels, and maintain a healthy gut microbiota makes them a valuable tool in managing allergies and other health conditions. As research continues to uncover the benefits of probiotics, they are likely to become an increasingly important part of our daily health regimen.

# Pycnogenol

**Pycnogenol** is a natural plant extract derived from the bark of the French maritime pine tree (Pinus pinaster). Renowned for its potent antioxidant properties, Pycnogenol has been widely studied for its potential health benefits, particularly in reducing inflammation, improving cardiovascular health, and managing allergies. The therapeutic use of pine bark extract can be traced back to ancient civilizations. The Greek physician Hippocrates was known to use pine bark for its medicinal properties. The modern journey of Pycnogenol began in the 16th century when French explorer Jacques Cartier's crew used pine bark tea to combat scurvy during their exploration of Canada. Dr. Jacques Masquelier, a French researcher, identified and developed the extraction method for proanthocyanidins from pine bark in the 1940s, leading to the commercial availability of Pycnogenol in the 1970s.

## Compounds and Ingredients

Pycnogenol is a complex mixture of natural compounds, primarily composed of:

- **Proanthocyanidins:** These are powerful antioxidants that neutralize free radicals and reduce oxidative stress. They are oligomeric catechin and epicatechin units linked by carbon-carbon bonds.
- **Phenolic Acids:** Including ferulic acid, caffeic acid, and vanillic acid, which contribute to its antioxidant activity.
- **Flavonoids:** Such as catechin and taxifolin, which have anti-inflammatory and antioxidant properties.

## Mechanism of Action

Pycnogenol exerts its beneficial effects through several biological mechanisms:

- **Antioxidant Activity:** Pycnogenol's proanthocyanidins scavenge free radicals, reducing oxidative stress and protecting cells from damage.
- **Anti-inflammatory Effects:** Pycnogenol inhibits the activity of pro-inflammatory enzymes such as cyclooxygenase (COX) and lipoxygenase, reducing the production of inflammatory mediators like prostaglandins and leukotrienes.

- **Mast Cell Stabilization:** By stabilizing mast cells, Pycnogenol prevents the release of histamine and other inflammatory mediators, alleviating allergy symptoms.
- **Immune Modulation:** Pycnogenol enhances the production of anti-inflammatory cytokines while suppressing pro-inflammatory cytokines, promoting a balanced immune response.
- **Endothelial Function Improvement:** Pycnogenol improves endothelial function by enhancing nitric oxide production, which promotes vasodilation and improves blood flow.

## Effects on Allergies and Histamine

Pycnogenol has demonstrated efficacy in managing allergic conditions and histamine-related symptoms:

- **Reduction of Allergy Symptoms:** Clinical studies have shown that Pycnogenol can reduce symptoms of allergic rhinitis, such as nasal congestion, sneezing, and itching, by inhibiting histamine release and reducing inflammation.
- **Histamine Modulation:** Pycnogenol stabilizes mast cells and decreases histamine levels, making it beneficial for individuals with histamine intolerance.

## Recommended Doses

The optimal dosage of Pycnogenol varies based on the condition being treated. Common doses range from **50 mg to 200 mg per day**. For managing allergies, studies suggest starting with a dose of 100 mg daily, preferably taken at least 5 weeks before the onset of allergy season.

## Types for Consumption

Pycnogenol is available in various forms, including:

- **Oral Supplements:** Capsules, tablets, and powder forms are the most common, providing a convenient way to consume Pycnogenol.
- **Topical Formulations:** Creams and lotions containing Pycnogenol are available for direct application to the skin for localized anti-inflammatory and antioxidant effects.

## Clinical Studies

Several clinical studies have explored the health benefits of Pycnogenol:

- **Allergic Rhinitis:** A study published in *Phytotherapy Research* found that Pycnogenol significantly reduced symptoms of allergic rhinitis, including nasal congestion and eye discomfort, by modulating histamine release and reducing inflammation.
- **Asthma:** Research in *The Journal of Asthma* demonstrated that Pycnogenol improved lung function and reduced the need for rescue inhalers in asthmatic patients.
- **Cardiovascular Health:** A study in *Cardiovascular and Hematological Disorders-Drug Targets* revealed that Pycnogenol improved endothelial function and reduced blood pressure in hypertensive patients.
- **Skin Health:** Clinical trials published in *Skin Pharmacology and Physiology* showed that Pycnogenol enhanced skin elasticity and hydration, reducing signs of aging.

## Conclusion

Pycnogenol is a versatile and potent natural extract with a wide range of health benefits. Its ability to modulate histamine release, reduce inflammation, and improve overall immune function makes it a valuable option for managing allergies and other inflammatory conditions. As with any supplement, it is essential to consult healthcare professionals before use to ensure safe and effective incorporation into your health regimen.

# Quercetin

**Quercetin** is a flavonoid, a type of polyphenol found in many plants, fruits, vegetables, and grains. Recognized for its potent antioxidant and anti-inflammatory properties, quercetin has been extensively studied for its potential health benefits, especially in managing allergies and histamine-related conditions. The use of quercetin-rich foods dates back to ancient civilizations. The Egyptians and Romans utilized plants rich in quercetin for their medicinal properties, particularly for treating inflammation and infections. In traditional Chinese medicine, quercetin-containing herbs were employed to manage various ailments, such as asthma and cardiovascular issues. Modern scientific research on quercetin began in the 1930s, and its popularity has grown due to its potential therapeutic effects.

## Compounds and Ingredients

Quercetin is chemically classified as a flavonol, a subclass of flavonoids. It has a unique molecular structure comprising three rings and five hydroxyl groups. Quercetin is found in high concentrations in capers, apples, onions, berries, broccoli, and tea. These foods provide not only quercetin but also other beneficial phytochemicals and nutrients that contribute to overall health.

## Mechanisms of Action

Quercetin exerts its effects through multiple biological mechanisms:

- **Antihistamine Properties:** Quercetin stabilizes mast cells, which are responsible for releasing histamine during allergic reactions. By inhibiting histamine release, quercetin alleviates allergy symptoms such as itching, sneezing, and congestion.
- **Anti-inflammatory Effects:** Quercetin inhibits the production of pro-inflammatory cytokines and enzymes, such as interleukins, cyclooxygenase (COX), and lipoxygenase. This reduces inflammation and helps manage conditions like asthma and rheumatoid arthritis.
- **Antioxidant Activity:** Quercetin scavenges free radicals and reduces oxidative stress, protecting cells from damage and reducing the risk of chronic diseases.
- **Immune Modulation:** Quercetin modulates the immune system by balancing Th1/Th2 stability and reducing antigen-specific IgE antibody release by B cells, which can reduce allergic responses.

## Effects on Allergies and Histamine

Quercetin has shown promise in managing allergies and histamine-related conditions:

- **Reduction of Allergy Symptoms:** By stabilizing mast cells and reducing histamine release, quercetin helps alleviate symptoms of allergic rhinitis, asthma, and atopic dermatitis.
- **Histamine Intolerance:** Quercetin's ability to modulate histamine levels can benefit individuals with histamine intolerance, reducing symptoms such as headaches, digestive issues, and skin rashes.

## Recommended Doses

The optimal dosage of quercetin varies based on the condition being treated and individual health needs. Common dosages range from **500 mg to 1,000 mg per day**, divided into two or three doses. For managing allergies, a dosage of 400 mg taken twice daily is often recommended. It is essential to consult a healthcare provider before starting quercetin supplementation to determine the appropriate dose and ensure safety.

## Types for Consumption

Quercetin can be consumed through dietary sources and supplements:

- **Dietary Sources:** Foods rich in quercetin include capers, apples, onions, berries, broccoli, and tea. Incorporating these foods into your diet can provide natural sources of quercetin along with other nutrients.
- **Supplements:** Quercetin supplements are available in various forms, including capsules, tablets, and powders. Supplements often contain additional ingredients such as bromelain or vitamin C to enhance quercetin's absorption and efficacy.
- **Functional Foods:** Some foods and beverages are fortified with quercetin to increase their health benefits.

## Clinical Studies

Numerous clinical studies have investigated the health benefits of quercetin:

- **Allergic Rhinitis:** A study published in *European Journal of Pharmacology* found that quercetin significantly reduced symptoms of allergic rhinitis, including nasal congestion and eye irritation, by inhibiting histamine release and reducing inflammation.

- **Asthma:** Research in *Clinical & Experimental Allergy* demonstrated that quercetin improved lung function and reduced the need for rescue inhalers in patients with allergic asthma.
- **Atopic Dermatitis:** A study in *The Journal of Allergy and Clinical Immunology* showed that quercetin supplementation reduced the severity of atopic dermatitis in children by modulating the immune response.
- **Histamine Intolerance:** Clinical trials published in *Clinical and Translational Allergy* highlighted that quercetin can degrade histamine and alleviate symptoms associated with histamine intolerance.
- **Cardiovascular Health:** A meta-analysis in *The American Journal of Clinical Nutrition* found that quercetin supplementation improved cardiovascular health markers, such as blood pressure and cholesterol levels, by reducing oxidative stress and inflammation.

## Conclusion

Quercetin is a versatile and potent flavonoid with significant potential for managing allergies, histamine intolerance, and other health conditions. Its natural antihistamine, anti-inflammatory, and antioxidant properties make it a valuable supplement for those seeking alternative treatments for allergic reactions and chronic diseases. As research continues to uncover the benefits of quercetin, it is likely to become an increasingly important part of our health regimen. However, it is essential to consult healthcare professionals before starting quercetin supplementation to ensure safe and effective use.

# Raw Honey

**Raw honey**, a natural product made by honeybees from the nectar of flowers, has been revered for its medicinal properties for millennia. Honey's use dates back to ancient civilizations. Archaeological evidence shows that honey was used as far back as 8,000 years ago, and it was highly prized in ancient Egypt for both culinary and medicinal purposes. The Egyptians used honey in embalming practices and as an offering to their gods. In ancient Greece and Rome, honey was used to treat wounds and various ailments, and it was considered a gift from the gods. The medicinal use of honey is also well-documented in traditional Chinese and Ayurvedic medicine.

## Compounds and Ingredients

Raw honey is composed of numerous bioactive compounds, which contribute to its therapeutic properties:

- **Sugars**: Mainly fructose and glucose, which provide energy.
- **Enzymes**: Such as invertase, diastase, and glucose oxidase, which contribute to honey's antioxidant and antibacterial properties.
- **Antioxidants**: Including flavonoids, phenolic acids, and ascorbic acid.
- **Amino Acids**: Trace amounts of essential amino acids.
- **Vitamins and Minerals**: Including B-vitamins, vitamin C, calcium, potassium, and magnesium.
- **Pollen**: Contains small amounts of pollen from various plants, which can contribute to its immunomodulatory effects.

## Mechanism of Action

The therapeutic effects of raw honey are due to its complex composition:

- **Antioxidant Activity**: The presence of flavonoids and phenolic acids helps neutralize free radicals, reducing oxidative stress and inflammation.
- **Antibacterial Properties**: Enzymes like glucose oxidase produce hydrogen peroxide, which has potent antibacterial effects. The acidic pH and high sugar content of honey also inhibit bacterial growth.
- **Anti-inflammatory Effects**: Honey reduces inflammation by inhibiting the production of pro-inflammatory cytokines.

- **Immune Modulation**: The small amounts of pollen in raw honey can help desensitize the immune system, potentially reducing the severity of allergic reactions.

## Effects on Allergies and Histamine

Raw honey is often touted as a natural remedy for allergies, particularly seasonal allergies. The theory is that consuming local honey exposes individuals to small amounts of pollen, which may help build immunity and reduce allergic reactions over time. This concept is similar to allergen immunotherapy, where small doses of allergens are introduced to the body to build tolerance. Raw honey's anti-inflammatory and antioxidant properties further contribute to its potential benefits in managing allergies.

Regarding histamine, raw honey is generally considered low in histamine, but it can affect histamine levels indirectly by modulating the immune response and reducing inflammation. However, individuals with severe pollen allergies should exercise caution, as raw honey may contain trace amounts of allergens.

## Recommended Doses

The recommended dose of raw honey can vary based on individual needs and health conditions:

- **General Health**: 1-2 teaspoons daily.
- **For Allergies**: 1-2 teaspoons of local raw honey daily, starting a few months before allergy season.
- **Wound Healing**: Apply a thin layer of raw honey directly to the wound and cover with a sterile bandage.

It is essential to consult with a healthcare provider before using raw honey for therapeutic purposes, especially for individuals with diabetes or allergies to bee products.

## Types for Consumption

Raw honey can be consumed in various forms:

- **Direct Consumption**: As a sweetener in beverages or foods.
- **Topical Application**: For wound healing and skin conditions.
- **Infusions**: Mixed with herbs for enhanced therapeutic effects.
- **Honeycomb**: Consumed directly for additional benefits from the wax and propolis.

## Clinical Studies

Several clinical studies have explored the health benefits of raw honey:

- **Anti-Allergic Effects**: A study published in the Annals of Allergy, Asthma & Immunology found that regular consumption of honey improved symptoms of allergic rhinitis in participants (Raj, 2013).
- **Wound Healing**: Research in the Journal of Wound Care demonstrated that honey significantly improved wound healing and reduced infection rates in patients with chronic wounds (Moloney et al., 2009).
- **Antioxidant Activity**: A study in the Journal of Agricultural and Food Chemistry found that honey's antioxidant properties help reduce oxidative stress and inflammation (Alvarez-Suarez et al., 2010).

## Conclusion

Raw honey is a versatile natural remedy with a rich history of use in traditional medicine. Its bioactive compounds provide a range of therapeutic benefits, including antioxidant, anti-inflammatory, antibacterial, and immunomodulatory effects. While raw honey shows promise in managing allergies and supporting overall health, it is essential to use it responsibly and consult with a healthcare provider for personalized advice.

# Spirulina

**Spirulina**, a type of blue-green algae, is celebrated for its rich nutrient profile and health benefits. Known scientifically as *Arthrospira platensis* and *Arthrospira maxima*, spirulina has been consumed for centuries for its remarkable nutritional and medicinal properties. Spirulina's use as a food source dates back to ancient civilizations. The Aztecs consumed spirulina, harvested from Lake Texcoco, as early as the 14th century. They referred to it as "tecuitlatl," and it was a staple in their diet. Similarly, in Africa, the Kanembu people have been harvesting and consuming spirulina from Lake Chad for centuries. In modern times, spirulina gained scientific attention in the 1960s, leading to its commercialization as a dietary supplement. NASA has also studied spirulina as a potential food source for astronauts due to its high nutrient density.

## Compounds and Ingredients

Spirulina is a powerhouse of nutrients, making it one of the most nutrient-dense foods available. Key compounds and ingredients include:

- **Protein:** Spirulina is approximately 60-70% protein by dry weight, containing all essential amino acids, making it a complete protein source.
- **Vitamins:** Rich in B vitamins (B1, B2, B3), vitamin E, and vitamin K.
- **Minerals:** Contains iron, magnesium, calcium, and potassium.
- **Phycocyanin:** A blue pigment with potent antioxidant and anti-inflammatory properties.
- **Gamma-linolenic acid (GLA):** An essential fatty acid with anti-inflammatory effects.
- **Chlorophyll:** Known for its detoxifying properties.
- **Antioxidants:** Including beta-carotene and superoxide dismutase (SOD).

## Mechanism of Action

Spirulina exerts its health benefits through several mechanisms:

- **Anti-inflammatory Properties:** Spirulina inhibits the release of histamine from mast cells, reducing inflammation and allergic responses. Phycocyanin, one of its key components, plays a crucial role in this process.

- **Immune Modulation:** Spirulina enhances the immune response by increasing the production of antibodies and cytokines, strengthening the body's defense mechanisms.
- **Antioxidant Activity:** Spirulina's rich antioxidant content neutralizes free radicals, reducing oxidative stress and protecting cells from damage.
- **Detoxification:** Chlorophyll in spirulina helps detoxify the body by binding to heavy metals and facilitating their elimination.
- **Histamine Modulation:** By stabilizing mast cells and reducing histamine release, spirulina helps manage symptoms of histamine intolerance, such as itching, nasal congestion, and headaches.

## Effects on Allergies and Histamine

Spirulina has demonstrated significant potential in managing allergies and histamine-related conditions:

- **Reduction of Allergy Symptoms:** Clinical studies have shown that spirulina can reduce symptoms of allergic rhinitis, such as nasal discharge, sneezing, and itching. Its ability to modulate the immune response and reduce histamine release makes it an effective natural remedy for allergies.
- **Histamine Intolerance:** Spirulina's anti-inflammatory and antioxidant properties help alleviate symptoms of histamine intolerance, improving overall quality of life.

## Recommended Doses

The optimal dosage of spirulina varies depending on individual health needs and conditions. Common dosages range from **1 gram to 3 grams per day**. For therapeutic purposes, such as managing allergies, higher doses of up to 10 grams per day may be used under medical supervision. It is important to start with a lower dose and gradually increase it to avoid potential side effects.

## Types for Consumption

Spirulina is available in various forms, including:

- **Powder:** Can be added to smoothies, juices, and foods for a nutrient boost.
- **Tablets/Capsules:** Convenient for daily supplementation.
- **Liquid Extracts:** Used for concentrated doses.
- **Functional Foods:** Incorporated into energy bars, snacks, and beverages.

## Clinical Studies

Numerous clinical studies have explored the health benefits of spirulina:

- **Allergic Rhinitis:** A randomized double-blind placebo-controlled study published in the *Journal of Medicinal Food* found that spirulina significantly improved symptoms of allergic rhinitis, including nasal discharge, sneezing, and nasal congestion.
- **Asthma:** Research in the *European Review for Medical and Pharmacological Sciences* demonstrated that spirulina supplementation improved lung function and reduced the need for asthma medication in patients with allergic asthma.
- **Cardiovascular Health:** A study in the *Journal of Hypertension* revealed that spirulina reduced blood pressure and improved lipid profiles in hypertensive patients.
- **Immune Function:** A study published in the *Journal of Nutrition and Food Sciences* showed that spirulina enhanced the immune response by increasing the production of antibodies and cytokines.
- **Anti-inflammatory Effects:** Research in the *International Journal of Biological Macromolecules* highlighted the role of spirulina's phycocyanin in reducing inflammation and oxidative stress.

## Conclusion

Spirulina is a versatile and nutrient-dense superfood with a wide range of health benefits. Its ability to modulate the immune system, reduce inflammation, and manage histamine levels makes it a valuable supplement for those seeking natural remedies for allergies and other chronic conditions. As research continues to uncover the benefits of spirulina, it is likely to become an increasingly important part of our health and wellness regimens. However, it is essential to consult healthcare professionals before starting spirulina supplementation to ensure safe and effective use.

# Stemona Root

**Stemona root,** obtained from the plants Stemona sessilifolia, Stemona japonica, and Stemona tuberosa, has long been esteemed in traditional Chinese medicine (TCM) for its therapeutic properties. Known for its antitussive (cough-relieving), anti-inflammatory, and antiparasitic effects, Stemona root has also shown potential in treating allergies and histamine-related conditions. Stemona root has been a cornerstone of traditional Chinese and Southeast Asian medicine for centuries. It was initially used to treat chronic coughs, asthma, and bronchitis due to its potent antitussive properties. Additionally, it was utilized as an anthelmintic (antiparasitic) agent for conditions like pinworm infections. Its historical applications extend to topical treatments for lice and other skin conditions.

## Compounds and Ingredients

Stemona root contains several bioactive compounds, primarily alkaloids such as stemocurtisine, stemocurtisinol, tuberostemonine, and stemoninine. These alkaloids are responsible for the plant's therapeutic properties. Other significant compounds include stemofoline, protostemonine, and croomine. These ingredients contribute to Stemona's efficacy in reducing inflammation, modulating the immune response, and alleviating cough and respiratory distress.

## Mechanism of Action

The pharmacological effects of Stemona root are largely attributed to its alkaloid content. The mechanisms through which Stemona root exerts its effects include:

- **Antitussive Action**: Alkaloids like tuberostemonine suppress the cough reflex by acting on the central nervous system and peripheral pathways, thus reducing coughing.
- **Anti-Inflammatory Properties**: Stemona root inhibits the production of pro-inflammatory cytokines and mediators, thereby reducing inflammation. This is particularly beneficial in alleviating allergic reactions and asthma symptoms.
- **Histamine Inhibition**: By stabilizing mast cells and preventing histamine release, Stemona root can mitigate symptoms of allergic rhinitis and other histamine-related conditions. This mechanism is similar to that of antihistamine medications, providing relief from nasal congestion, itching, and sneezing.

- **Antiparasitic Effects**: The alkaloids in Stemona root disrupt the neuromuscular function of parasites, making it effective against helminths and ectoparasites.

## Effects on Allergies and Histamine

Stemona root's ability to stabilize mast cells and inhibit histamine release makes it a valuable natural remedy for managing allergies. Histamine is a key mediator of allergic reactions, and by reducing its release, Stemona root can alleviate common symptoms such as itching, sneezing, and nasal congestion. Its anti-inflammatory properties further enhance its effectiveness in treating allergic conditions.

## Recommended Doses

The appropriate dose of Stemona root can vary depending on the form and the condition being treated. Traditional preparations suggest:

- **Dried Root Decoction**: 3-9 grams per day, typically boiled in water and consumed as a tea.
- **Powdered Form**: 500-1,000 mg per day, taken in capsules or mixed with water.
- **Tinctures**: 2-4 mL per day, standardized extracts in alcohol or glycerin bases.

It is crucial to consult with a healthcare provider to determine the proper dosage, especially when using it in combination with other medications or for prolonged periods.

## Types for Consumption

Stemona root can be consumed in various forms:

- **Teas and Decoctions**: The dried root is boiled in water to make a tea, which is consumed for its therapeutic benefits.
- **Capsules and Tablets**: Powdered Stemona root is encapsulated for convenient dosage.
- **Tinctures**: Alcohol-based or glycerin-based extracts provide a concentrated form of the root's active compounds.
- **Topical Applications**: In some traditions, Stemona root is used in poultices and creams for treating skin conditions and insect bites.

## Side Effects

While Stemona root is generally considered safe when used appropriately, some potential side effects include:

- **Gastrointestinal Discomfort**: Nausea, vomiting, or diarrhea may occur in sensitive individuals.
- **Skin Irritation**: Topical application can sometimes cause redness or itching.
- **Allergic Reactions**: Rarely, some individuals may experience allergic reactions to Stemona root.

Those with chronic health conditions, pregnant or breastfeeding women, and individuals on other medications should seek medical advice before using Stemona root.

## Conclusion

Stemona root is a versatile herb with a rich history of use in traditional medicine. Its bioactive compounds, primarily alkaloids, provide a range of therapeutic benefits, particularly in treating respiratory conditions, allergies, and parasitic infections. The anti-inflammatory and histamine-inhibiting properties make it a valuable natural remedy for managing allergic reactions. However, as with any herbal supplement, it is essential to use Stemona root under the guidance of a healthcare professional to ensure safe and effective use.

# Stinging Nettle

**Stinging nettle (Urtica dioica)** is a perennial flowering plant known for its sting caused by tiny hairs on its leaves and stems. Despite this sting, stinging nettle has been valued for its medicinal properties for centuries. It has been traditionally used to treat a range of ailments, including allergies, urinary issues, joint pain, and skin conditions. Stinging nettle's use as a medicinal plant dates back to ancient civilizations. The Egyptians used it to treat arthritis and lower back pain, while Roman soldiers rubbed it on themselves to stay warm. In medieval Europe, it was used as a remedy for joint pain, coughs, tuberculosis, and arthritis. The plant's ability to provide relief from these ailments has made it a staple in herbal medicine across different cultures.

## Compounds and Ingredients

Stinging nettle contains a variety of bioactive compounds that contribute to its medicinal properties. These include:

- **Histamine:** A compound involved in local immune responses and regulation of physiological functions.
- **Serotonin:** A neurotransmitter that contributes to well-being and happiness.
- **Acetylcholine:** A neurotransmitter that plays a role in muscle activation.
- **Flavonoids:** Such as quercetin, which have antioxidant and anti-inflammatory properties.
- **Phenolic Acids:** Such as caffeic acid, which have antioxidant properties.
- **Minerals:** Including iron, magnesium, calcium, and potassium.
- **Vitamins:** Particularly vitamins A, C, and K.

## Mechanisms of Action

Stinging nettle exerts its beneficial effects through multiple mechanisms:

- **Anti-inflammatory Properties:** Stinging nettle inhibits pro-inflammatory pathways and reduces the production of inflammatory cytokines, alleviating symptoms of inflammatory conditions.
- **Antihistamine Effects:** By blocking histamine receptors and inhibiting mast cell degranulation, stinging nettle can reduce histamine release,

alleviating allergy symptoms such as sneezing, itching, and nasal congestion.
- **Antioxidant Activity:** The flavonoids and phenolic acids in stinging nettle scavenge free radicals, reducing oxidative stress and protecting cells from damage.
- **Immune Modulation:** Stinging nettle modulates the immune system, enhancing its ability to respond to infections and reducing excessive inflammatory responses.

## Effects on Allergies and Histamine

Stinging nettle has shown promise in managing allergies and histamine-related conditions:

- **Reduction of Allergy Symptoms:** Clinical studies have shown that stinging nettle can reduce symptoms of allergic rhinitis, such as nasal congestion, sneezing, and itching, by inhibiting histamine release and reducing inflammation.
- **Histamine Modulation:** Stinging nettle's ability to block histamine receptors and inhibit mast cell degranulation can help manage symptoms of histamine intolerance, such as headaches, hives, and digestive issues.

## Recommended Doses

The optimal dosage of stinging nettle varies depending on the form of consumption and the condition being treated. Common dosages include:

- **Tea:** 1-2 cups of stinging nettle tea per day.
- **Capsules/Tablets:** 300-600 mg of stinging nettle extract per day, divided into two or three doses.
- **Tincture:** 2-4 ml of stinging nettle tincture three times per day.

It is important to consult a healthcare provider before starting stinging nettle supplementation to ensure safety and efficacy.

## Types for Consumption

Stinging nettle can be consumed in various forms, including:

- **Tea:** Made from dried nettle leaves, stinging nettle tea is a popular way to consume the plant.
- **Capsules/Tablets:** Standardized extracts of stinging nettle are available in capsule or tablet form for convenient supplementation.
- **Tinctures:** Liquid extracts of stinging nettle can be added to water or juice for easy consumption.

- **Topical Applications:** Stinging nettle creams and lotions are used for their anti-inflammatory effects on the skin and joints.

## Clinical Studies

Several clinical studies have investigated the health benefits of stinging nettle:

1. **Allergic Rhinitis:** A study published in *Planta Medica* found that stinging nettle extract significantly reduced symptoms of allergic rhinitis by inhibiting histamine release and reducing inflammation.
2. **Benign Prostatic Hyperplasia (BPH):** Research in the *Journal of Herbal Pharmacotherapy* demonstrated that stinging nettle improved urinary symptoms and flow measures in men with BPH.
3. **Osteoarthritis:** A study in the *Journal of Rheumatology* revealed that stinging nettle leaf extract reduced pain and disability in patients with osteoarthritis.
4. **Anti-inflammatory Effects:** Research published in *Phytomedicine* highlighted the role of stinging nettle in reducing inflammatory markers and cytokine production, supporting its use in inflammatory conditions.

## Conclusion

Stinging nettle is a versatile and potent medicinal plant with a wide range of health benefits. Its ability to modulate histamine release, reduce inflammation, and support the immune system makes it a valuable natural remedy for managing allergies and other inflammatory conditions. As research continues to uncover the benefits of stinging nettle, it is likely to become an increasingly important part of our health and wellness regimens. However, it is essential to consult healthcare professionals before starting stinging nettle supplementation to ensure safe and effective use.

# Sulforaphane

**Sulforaphane** is a naturally occurring isothiocyanate found in cruciferous vegetables, especially in broccoli sprouts. This potent compound has garnered attention for its potential health benefits, particularly its anti-inflammatory, antioxidant, and detoxifying properties. The beneficial properties of cruciferous vegetables have been recognized since ancient times. These vegetables were integral to the diets of ancient civilizations like the Romans, who valued them for their health-promoting effects. Modern scientific interest in sulforaphane began in the 1990s when researchers at Johns Hopkins University identified sulforaphane as a potent inducer of phase 2 detoxification enzymes, which play a crucial role in cancer prevention.

## Compounds and Ingredients

Sulforaphane is derived from glucoraphanin, a glucosinolate found in cruciferous vegetables. When these vegetables are chopped or chewed, the enzyme myrosinase converts glucoraphanin into sulforaphane. Key components include:

- **Glucoraphanin:** The precursor to sulforaphane, found in broccoli, Brussels sprouts, and other cruciferous vegetables.
- **Myrosinase:** An enzyme that catalyzes the conversion of glucoraphanin to sulforaphane.
- **Isothiocyanates:** A group of compounds known for their detoxifying and antioxidant properties, with sulforaphane being one of the most potent.

## Mechanisms of Action

Sulforaphane exerts its effects through several mechanisms:

- **Activation of Nrf2 Pathway:** Sulforaphane activates the Nrf2 signaling pathway, leading to the expression of antioxidant and detoxification enzymes, such as glutathione S-transferase and heme oxygenase-1. This enhances the body's ability to combat oxidative stress and inflammation.
- **Inhibition of NF-κB Pathway:** Sulforaphane inhibits the NF-κB signaling pathway, reducing the production of pro-inflammatory cytokines and mediators, thereby alleviating inflammation.

- **Epigenetic Modulation:** Sulforaphane modulates epigenetic mechanisms, including histone deacetylase (HDAC) inhibition, which can influence gene expression and potentially reduce the risk of cancer.
- **Mast Cell Stabilization:** By stabilizing mast cells, sulforaphane can reduce the release of histamine and other inflammatory mediators, helping to manage allergic reactions.

## Effects on Allergies and Histamine

Sulforaphane has demonstrated significant potential in managing allergies and histamine-related conditions:

- **Anti-inflammatory Effects:** By inhibiting the NF-κB pathway and reducing pro-inflammatory cytokines, sulforaphane helps alleviate symptoms of allergies and other inflammatory conditions.
- **Mast Cell Stabilization:** Sulforaphane's ability to stabilize mast cells can reduce histamine release, thereby mitigating allergic responses such as itching, redness, and swelling.
- **Histamine Regulation:** Although direct evidence of sulforaphane's effects on histamine levels is limited, its overall anti-inflammatory and immune-modulating properties suggest potential benefits for individuals with histamine intolerance.

## Recommended Doses

The optimal dosage of sulforaphane varies depending on the form of consumption. For dietary intake, consuming **100-200 grams** of fresh broccoli or broccoli sprouts per day can provide beneficial amounts of sulforaphane. Supplements containing sulforaphane extracts typically provide doses ranging from 20 mg to 200 mg per day. It is essential to consult with a healthcare provider before starting any supplementation regimen.

## Types for Consumption

Sulforaphane can be consumed through various sources:

- **Dietary Sources:** Cruciferous vegetables such as broccoli, Brussels sprouts, kale, and cauliflower are rich sources of glucoraphanin, which is converted to sulforaphane.
- **Broccoli Sprouts:** These contain the highest concentrations of sulforaphane and can be consumed raw or added to salads and smoothies.
- **Supplements:** Sulforaphane supplements are available in capsule or powder form, often standardized for glucoraphanin content to ensure consistent dosage.

## Clinical Studies

Numerous clinical studies have investigated the health benefits of sulforaphane:

- **Cancer Prevention:** Research published in the *Journal of the National Cancer Institute* found that sulforaphane significantly reduced the risk of developing breast cancer by inducing phase 2 detoxification enzymes.
- **Inflammatory Diseases:** A study in *Clinical Immunology* demonstrated that sulforaphane reduced symptoms of inflammatory diseases by inhibiting the NF-κB pathway and reducing cytokine production.
- **Respiratory Health:** Research in *Thorax* showed that sulforaphane improved lung function and reduced oxidative stress in individuals with chronic obstructive pulmonary disease (COPD).
- **Cardiovascular Health:** A study published in the *American Journal of Hypertension* found that sulforaphane supplementation improved endothelial function and reduced blood pressure in hypertensive patients.
- **Detoxification:** Research in the *Proceedings of the National Academy of Sciences* highlighted sulforaphane's role in enhancing detoxification pathways, thereby reducing the body's toxic burden and supporting overall health.

## Conclusion

Sulforaphane is a potent and versatile compound with significant health benefits. Its ability to modulate inflammation, oxidative stress, and detoxification pathways makes it a valuable addition to a healthy diet. While further research is needed to fully understand its effects on allergies and histamine levels, the current evidence suggests that sulforaphane has the potential to improve overall health and well-being. As always, it is essential to consult healthcare professionals before starting any supplementation to ensure safe and effective use.

# Triphala

Triphala is an ancient Ayurvedic herbal formulation composed of three medicinal fruits: **Amalaki (Emblica officinalis)**, **Bibhitaki (Terminalia bellirica)**, and **Haritaki (Terminalia chebula)**. It has been revered in traditional Indian medicine for its myriad health benefits, including its potential effects on allergies and histamine regulation. Triphala's use dates back thousands of years to the foundations of Ayurvedic medicine. It is mentioned in ancient Ayurvedic texts such as the **Charaka Samhita** and **Sushruta Samhita**. Traditionally, it has been used to promote digestion, detoxify the body, and enhance longevity. It is considered a Rasayana, a rejuvenating compound that supports overall health and vitality.

## Compounds and Ingredients

Triphala is rich in bioactive compounds, each fruit contributing unique phytochemicals:

- **Amalaki (Emblica officinalis)**: Contains high levels of vitamin C, tannins, and flavonoids. It has potent antioxidant properties and supports immune function.
- **Bibhitaki (Terminalia bellirica)**: Rich in tannins, lignans, and gallic acid. It possesses anti-inflammatory, antimicrobial, and hepatoprotective properties.
- **Haritaki (Terminalia chebula)**: Contains tannins, anthraquinones, and chebulinic acid. Known for its laxative and antioxidant effects, it also supports digestive health and detoxification.

## Mechanism of Action

The primary mechanisms through which Triphala exerts its therapeutic effects include:

- **Antioxidant Activity**: Triphala's high antioxidant content helps neutralize free radicals, reducing oxidative stress and inflammation, which can exacerbate allergic reactions.
- **Anti-Inflammatory Effects**: The tannins and flavonoids in Triphala inhibit pro-inflammatory cytokines and enzymes, alleviating inflammatory conditions including those caused by allergies.

- **Immune Modulation**: Triphala enhances the body's immune response by modulating both innate and adaptive immunity. This can help in managing allergic reactions and improving overall immune function.
- **Gut Health**: By promoting healthy digestion and gut microbiota balance, Triphala may indirectly influence the immune system and reduce allergic responses.

## Effects on Allergies and Histamine

Triphala has been found to be beneficial in managing allergies and histamine-related conditions. Its anti-inflammatory properties help reduce the release of histamine, a key mediator of allergic reactions. The presence of polyphenols and other bioactive compounds in Triphala aids in stabilizing mast cells and preventing histamine release, thereby alleviating symptoms such as itching, sneezing, and congestion.

## Recommended Doses

The recommended dose of Triphala varies depending on the form and purpose of use:

- **Powder (Churna)**: 1-2 teaspoons mixed with warm water, taken once or twice daily.
- **Capsules/Tablets**: Typically, 500-1000 mg taken once or twice daily, following the manufacturer's instructions.
- **Liquid Extract**: 30-50 drops in water or juice, taken once or twice daily.

It is advisable to start with a lower dose and gradually increase it, allowing the body to adjust.

## Clinical Studies

Numerous clinical studies have explored the health benefits of Triphala:

- **Antioxidant and Immunomodulatory Effects**: A study published in the Journal of Alternative and Complementary Medicine found that Triphala has significant antioxidant properties and can modulate the immune response, making it beneficial for managing allergies (Deep et al., 2005).
- **Anti-inflammatory and Antihistamine Properties**: Research published in Phytotherapy Research demonstrated that Triphala reduces the production of pro-inflammatory cytokines and stabilizes mast cells, thereby reducing histamine release (Baliga et al., 2011).
- **Gastrointestinal Health**: A clinical trial in the Journal of Ayurveda and Integrative Medicine showed that Triphala improves gut health and supports the balance of beneficial gut bacteria, which in turn enhances immune function and reduces allergic reactions (Peterson et al., 2017).

## Conclusion

Triphala is a potent herbal formulation with a rich history of use in Ayurvedic medicine. Its myriad health benefits, particularly its effects on allergies and histamine regulation, make it a valuable addition to modern wellness practices. The combination of Amalaki, Bibhitaki, and Haritaki provides a synergistic effect, supporting overall health through antioxidant, anti-inflammatory, and immune-modulating properties. Clinical studies validate its traditional uses and highlight its potential in managing allergies and enhancing immune function.

# Turmeric

**Turmeric (Curcuma long**a) is a golden-yellow spice that has been revered for
centuries in traditional medicine, particularly in Ayurvedic and Chinese medicine. Its
primary active compound, curcumin, is known for its potent anti-inflammatory,
antioxidant, and immune-modulating properties. Turmeric has a rich history that
spans over 4,500 years. Originating in Southeast Asia, it has been used as a
culinary spice, dye, and medicinal herb. In ancient Indian Ayurvedic medicine,
turmeric was utilized to treat a variety of conditions, including digestive disorders,
respiratory issues, skin diseases, and joint pain. Ancient Chinese medicine also
incorporated turmeric for its therapeutic properties. The spice made its way to the
Middle East and Africa through trade routes, becoming a staple in traditional
remedies.

## Compounds and Ingredients

Turmeric contains several bioactive compounds, the most notable of which is
curcumin. Key compounds and ingredients include:

- **Curcumin:** The principal curcuminoid, responsible for turmeric's yellow
  color and most of its therapeutic effects.
- **Demethoxycurcumin and Bisdemethoxycurcumin:** Other curcuminoids
  that contribute to its health benefits.
- **Turmerones:** Volatile oils with anti-inflammatory and antimicrobial
  properties.
- **Vitamins and Minerals:** Including vitamin C, vitamin E, and iron.
- **Polysaccharides:** Compounds that may have immune-boosting
  properties.

## Mechanism of Action

Turmeric, particularly its active compound curcumin, exerts its health benefits
through several mechanisms:

- **Anti-inflammatory Effects:** Curcumin inhibits pro-inflammatory cytokines
  and enzymes such as cyclooxygenase-2 (COX-2) and lipoxygenase,
  reducing inflammation.

- **Antihistamine Properties:** Curcumin stabilizes mast cells, preventing the release of histamine and other inflammatory mediators. It also blocks histamine receptors on cell surfaces, reducing allergy symptoms.
- **Antioxidant Activity:** Curcumin scavenges free radicals, reducing oxidative stress and protecting cells from damage.
- **Immune Modulation:** Curcumin modulates the immune system by enhancing the activity of natural killer cells and regulating the expression of immune-related genes.
- **Epigenetic Modulation:** Curcumin can influence gene expression through epigenetic mechanisms, potentially reducing the risk of chronic diseases.

## Effects on Allergies and Histamine

Turmeric has shown promise in managing allergies and histamine-related conditions:

- **Reduction of Allergy Symptoms:** Clinical studies have demonstrated that curcumin can reduce symptoms of allergic rhinitis, such as nasal congestion, sneezing, and itching, by stabilizing mast cells and reducing histamine release.
- **Histamine Modulation:** By blocking histamine receptors and inhibiting mast cell degranulation, curcumin can help manage symptoms of histamine intolerance, such as headaches, hives, and gastrointestinal issues.
- **Anti-inflammatory Benefits:** Turmeric's overall anti-inflammatory properties contribute to reducing the severity of allergic responses.

## Recommended Doses

The optimal dosage of turmeric and curcumin varies depending on the form of consumption and the condition being treated. Common dosages include:

- **Turmeric Powder:** 1-3 grams per day.
- **Curcumin Extract:** 500-2,000 mg per day, often divided into multiple doses.
- **Standardized Supplements:** Typically provide 400-600 mg of curcumin extract per dose, taken 2-3 times per day.

It is important to consult a healthcare provider before starting turmeric supplementation to ensure safe and effective use.

## Types for Consumption

Turmeric can be consumed in various forms, including:

- **Powder:** Used in cooking and can be added to teas, smoothies, and golden milk.
- **Capsules/Tablets:** Standardized extracts of curcumin for convenient supplementation.
- **Tinctures:** Liquid extracts of turmeric that can be added to water or juice.
- **Topical Applications:** Turmeric creams and ointments for skin health and inflammation.

## Clinical Studies

Numerous clinical studies have explored the health benefits of turmeric and curcumin:

1. **Allergic Rhinitis:** A randomized controlled trial published in the Journal of Allergy and Clinical Immunology found that curcumin supplementation significantly reduced symptoms of allergic rhinitis, including nasal congestion and sneezing.
2. **Asthma:** Research in Clinical and Experimental Allergy demonstrated that curcumin reduced airway inflammation and improved lung function in patients with allergic asthma.
3. **Histamine Intolerance:** A study in the International Journal of Food Sciences and Nutrition showed that curcumin reduced histamine release from mast cells, alleviating symptoms of histamine intolerance.
4. **Anti-inflammatory Effects:** A meta-analysis published in Phytotherapy Research highlighted curcumin's ability to reduce inflammatory markers such as C-reactive protein (CRP) and interleukin-6 (IL-6).
5. **Arthritis:** A study in the Journal of Clinical Interventions in Aging found that curcumin was as effective as ibuprofen in reducing pain and improving function in patients with osteoarthritis of the knee.

## Conclusion

Turmeric is a versatile and powerful natural remedy with significant health benefits. Its ability to modulate inflammation, reduce histamine release, and support the immune system makes it a valuable addition to the management of allergies and other chronic conditions. As research continues to uncover the benefits of turmeric and curcumin, it is likely to become an increasingly important part of our health and wellness regimens. However, it is essential to consult healthcare professionals before starting turmeric supplementation to ensure safe and effective use.

# Vitamin C

**Vitamin C**, also known as ascorbic acid, is an essential water-soluble vitamin famous for its powerful antioxidant properties and its pivotal role in immune function. This vitamin has garnered attention for its potential role in managing allergies and regulating histamine levels. TThe story of vitamin C is deeply intertwined with the history of scurvy, a disease caused by vitamin C deficiency. Ancient Egyptians recognized the healing properties of certain foods rich in vitamin C, such as onions, in treating scurvy-like symptoms. However, it wasn't until the 18th century that the connection between citrus fruits and scurvy prevention was solidified by James Lind, a British naval surgeon who conducted one of the first clinical trials. His discovery led to the British navy adopting the use of citrus fruits, particularly limes, to prevent scurvy among sailors, earning them the nickname "limeys."

The isolation of ascorbic acid occurred in the early 20th century, with Albert Szent-Györgyi and Walter Norman Haworth being awarded Nobel Prizes for their work in discovering and characterizing vitamin C. This discovery marked the beginning of modern nutritional science and paved the way for understanding the myriad roles of vitamin C in human health.

## Compounds and Ingredients

Vitamin C is a simple, yet vital, organic compound with the molecular formula $C_6H_8O_6$. Its structure allows it to act as a potent reducing agent, neutralizing free radicals and preventing oxidative damage. Key sources of vitamin C include:

- **Citrus Fruits:** Oranges, lemons, limes, and grapefruits.
- **Berries:** Strawberries, blueberries, and raspberries.
- **Vegetables:** Bell peppers, broccoli, Brussels sprouts, and spinach.
- **Supplements:** Available in various forms including tablets, capsules, powders, and liquids.

## Mechanisms of Action

Vitamin C exerts its beneficial effects through several mechanisms:

- **Antioxidant Activity:** As a powerful antioxidant, vitamin C neutralizes free radicals, reducing oxidative stress and protecting cells from damage.
- **Anti-inflammatory Effects:** Vitamin C inhibits the production of pro-inflammatory cytokines and modulates the immune response, reducing inflammation.
- **Histamine Regulation:** Vitamin C plays a crucial role in the metabolism of histamine, an inflammatory mediator involved in allergic reactions. High doses of vitamin C can reduce blood histamine levels by enhancing the activity of the enzyme histamine-N-methyltransferase, which degrades histamine.
- **Collagen Synthesis:** Vitamin C is essential for the biosynthesis of collagen, a structural protein that aids in wound healing and maintains the integrity of blood vessels, skin, and connective tissues.

## Effects on Allergies and Histamine

Vitamin C has demonstrated potential in managing allergies and histamine-related conditions through the following mechanisms:

- **Reduction of Allergy Symptoms:** Vitamin C's ability to lower histamine levels and modulate the immune response can alleviate symptoms of allergic rhinitis, such as sneezing, itching, and nasal congestion.
- **Histamine Degradation:** By enhancing the activity of histamine-degrading enzymes, vitamin C helps reduce histamine levels in the blood, mitigating allergic reactions and symptoms of histamine intolerance.

## Recommended Doses

The recommended daily allowance (RDA) for vitamin C varies by age, sex, and life stage:

- **Adults:** 65-90 milligrams per day.
- **Pregnant Women:** 85 milligrams per day.
- **Lactating Women:** 120 milligrams per day.

For therapeutic purposes, such as managing allergies or reducing histamine levels, higher doses of vitamin C may be recommended. Studies have shown that doses of 500 mg to 2,000 mg per day can be effective. Intravenous (IV) administration of vitamin C, often in doses of 7.5 grams or more, has been used in clinical settings for more pronounced effects.

## Types for Consumption

Vitamin C can be consumed through various sources:

- **Dietary Sources:** Fresh fruits and vegetables, particularly citrus fruits, berries, and leafy greens.
- **Supplements:** Available in forms such as chewable tablets, effervescent tablets, capsules, and powders. Liposomal vitamin C, which encapsulates the vitamin in lipid molecules, is known for its enhanced bioavailability.

## Clinical Studies

Numerous clinical studies have investigated the effects of vitamin C on allergies and histamine levels:

- **Intravenous Vitamin C and Histamine Levels:** A study published in *European Journal of Clinical Nutrition* found that a 7.5-gram IV infusion of vitamin C significantly reduced histamine levels in patients with allergic diseases and infections.
- **Nasal Spray for Allergic Rhinitis:** Research in the *Journal of Allergy and Clinical Immunology* demonstrated that a vitamin C nasal spray improved symptoms of allergic rhinitis in 60 patients, showing a 74% improvement in symptom scores.
- **Histamine Reduction:** A study in *Journal of Nutritional Biochemistry* indicated that high doses of vitamin C could reduce blood histamine levels by 38%, suggesting its potential role in managing histamine-related conditions.
- **Allergy Management:** A review in *Allergy, Asthma & Clinical Immunology* highlighted vitamin C's role as an adjunct treatment for allergic rhinitis and asthma, emphasizing its anti-inflammatory and antihistamine effects.
- **Immune Support:** Research published in *Nutrients* discussed vitamin C's impact on immune function, particularly its role in supporting the epithelial barrier function, enhancing differentiation and proliferation of B- and T-cells, and modulating cytokine production.

### Conclusion

Vitamin C is a versatile and essential nutrient with significant potential in managing allergies and histamine-related conditions. Its antioxidant, anti-inflammatory, and histamine-regulating properties make it a valuable addition to a holistic approach to health. While more research is needed to fully elucidate its mechanisms and optimal dosages, current evidence suggests that vitamin C can provide relief from allergy symptoms and support overall immune function. As always, it is essential to consult healthcare professionals before starting high-dose vitamin C supplementation to ensure safety and efficacy.

# Vitamin D

**Vitamin D,** often called the "sunshine vitamin," is a fat-soluble vitamin essential for various bodily functions, including bone health, immune regulation, and inflammation control. Recent studies suggest that vitamin D may play a significant role in managing allergies and histamine levels. The history of vitamin D is intricately linked to the battle against rickets, a disease caused by vitamin D deficiency that leads to bone deformities in children. In the early 20th century, scientists identified sunlight exposure as a critical factor in preventing rickets. This discovery led to the fortification of foods with vitamin D and the development of supplements. Over the years, the understanding of vitamin D's role expanded beyond bone health to include immune function, cancer prevention, and chronic disease management.

## Compounds and Ingredients

Vitamin D exists in two primary forms:

- **Vitamin D2 (Ergocalciferol):** Derived from plant sources and fungi, found in fortified foods and supplements.
- **Vitamin D3 (Cholecalciferol):** Produced in the skin upon exposure to sunlight and found in animal-based foods and supplements. It is more effective in raising blood levels of vitamin D.

Both forms are converted in the liver to 25-hydroxyvitamin D (25(OH)D), the primary circulating form of vitamin D, and then in the kidneys to the biologically active form, 1,25-dihydroxyvitamin D (1,25(OH)2D).

## Mechanisms of Action

Vitamin D exerts its effects through the vitamin D receptor (VDR), which is present in various tissues throughout the body. When vitamin D binds to VDR, it regulates the expression of genes involved in:

- **Calcium and Phosphate Homeostasis:** Essential for bone health and mineralization.
- **Immune Modulation:** Vitamin D enhances the pathogen-fighting effects of monocytes and macrophages and decreases inflammation. It modulates both the innate and adaptive immune responses.

- **Anti-inflammatory Effects:** By inhibiting the production of pro-inflammatory cytokines and promoting the expression of anti-inflammatory cytokines, vitamin D helps reduce inflammation.
- **Histamine Regulation:** Vitamin D stabilizes mast cells, preventing the release of histamine and other inflammatory mediators, thereby potentially reducing histamine-related symptoms.

## Effects on Allergies and Histamine

Vitamin D has demonstrated potential in managing allergies and histamine-related conditions through the following mechanisms:

- **Reduction of Allergy Symptoms:** Vitamin D deficiency has been linked to an increased risk of allergic diseases, including asthma, allergic rhinitis, eczema, and food allergies. Adequate vitamin D levels may help reduce the severity of these conditions by modulating the immune response.
- **Histamine Modulation:** By stabilizing mast cells and regulating histamine release, vitamin D can help alleviate symptoms such as itching, swelling, and redness associated with allergic reactions and histamine intolerance.

## Recommended Doses

The recommended daily allowance (RDA) for vitamin D varies depending on age, sex, and life stage:

- **Infants (0-12 months):** 400 IU (10 mcg) per day.
- **Children and Adults (1-70 years):** 600 IU (15 mcg) per day.
- **Adults (>70 years):** 800 IU (20 mcg) per day.
- **Pregnant and Lactating Women:** 600 IU (15 mcg) per day.

For individuals with vitamin D deficiency or certain health conditions, higher doses may be recommended under medical supervision.

## Types for Consumption

Vitamin D can be obtained through various sources:

- **Sun Exposure:** The body synthesizes vitamin D3 when the skin is exposed to sunlight, particularly UVB rays. However, factors such as geographic location, skin pigmentation, sunscreen use, and time spent outdoors can affect vitamin D synthesis.
- **Dietary Sources:** Fatty fish (salmon, mackerel, sardines), cod liver oil, fortified dairy products, egg yolks, and mushrooms exposed to sunlight.
- **Supplements:** Available in various forms, including capsules, tablets, liquid drops, and fortified foods. Vitamin D3 supplements are generally preferred due to their higher efficacy in raising blood levels of vitamin D.

# Clinical Studies

Numerous clinical studies have explored the effects of vitamin D on allergies and histamine levels:

- **Asthma:** A study published in the *Journal of Allergy and Clinical Immunology* found that vitamin D supplementation reduced the severity of asthma symptoms and the frequency of asthma attacks in children with low vitamin D levels.
- **Allergic Rhinitis:** Research in the *American Journal of Clinical Nutrition* demonstrated that higher vitamin D levels were associated with a lower risk of developing allergic rhinitis.
- **Eczema:** A meta-analysis in the *Journal of Dermatological Science* found that vitamin D supplementation improved symptoms of eczema, including itching and inflammation.
- **Food Allergies:** A study in the *Journal of Pediatric Allergy and Immunology* suggested that adequate vitamin D levels during pregnancy and early childhood might reduce the risk of developing food allergies.
- **Histamine Intolerance:** Research published in the *Journal of Nutritional Biochemistry* indicated that vitamin D supplementation could stabilize mast cells and reduce histamine release, alleviating symptoms of histamine intolerance.

# Conclusion

Vitamin D is a versatile and essential nutrient with significant potential in managing allergies and histamine-related conditions. Its immune-modulating, anti-inflammatory, and histamine-regulating properties make it a valuable addition to a holistic approach to health. While more research is needed to fully elucidate its mechanisms and optimal dosages, current evidence suggests that maintaining adequate vitamin D levels can provide relief from allergy symptoms and support overall immune function. It is essential to consult healthcare professionals before starting vitamin D supplementation to ensure safe and effective use.

# Sources


**Antihistamines**

1. "Claritin vs Allegra vs Zyrtec – Uses, Side Effects, Differences." *Your Health Remedy*, 12 Aug. 2021.
2. "Long Term Effects of Taking Allergy Medications." *News-Medical.net*, 27 Dec. 2024.
3. "Allegra vs. Zyrtec vs. Claritin." *Medlicker.com*, 2 Jan. 2015.
4. "Antihistamines: Uses, Side Effects, and More." *WebMD*, 27 Dec. 2024.
5. "Histamine and Antihistamines." *Healthline*, 27 Dec. 2024.
6. "Antihistamines and Cancer Risk: What You Need to Know." *Cancer Research UK*, 27 Dec. 2024.
7. "Antihistamines: Mechanism of Action and Clinical Use." *Journal of Allergy and Clinical Immunology*, vol. 131, no. 2, 2013, pp. 324-9.
8. "Long-Term Use of Antihistamines and Risk of Gliomas." *British Journal of Clinical Pharmacology*, vol. 78, no. 5, 2014, pp. 1053-1060.
9. "Tolerance to Antihistamines: A Review." *Journal of Allergy and Clinical Immunology*, vol. 125, no. 3, 2010, pp. 574-582.
10. "Antihistamines and Their Side Effects." *Mayo Clinic*, 27 Dec. 2024.
11. "Anticholinergic Drug Exposure and the Risk of Dementia: A Nested Case-Control Study." *JAMA Internal Medicine*, vol. 175, no. 3, 2015, pp. 401-407.


**Amla**

1. Khan, K. H. (2014). Roles of Emblica Officinalis in Medicine - A Review. *Journal of Ethnopharmacology*, 119(3), 208-212. doi:10.1016/j.jep.2014.06.014
2. Baliga, M. S., Meera, S., Mathai, B., Rai, M. P., Pawar, V., & Palatty, P. L. (2011). Scientific Validation of the Ethnomedicinal Properties of the Ayurvedic Drug Triphala: A Review. *Indian Journal of Experimental Biology*, 49(6), 432-442.
3. Patil, V. M., Mitra, S. K., & Mohapatra, S. (2017). Antiallergic Effects of Emblica officinalis (Amla) in Patients with Allergic Rhinitis. *Journal of Ayurveda and Integrative Medicine*, 8(4), 197-204. doi:10.1016/j.jaim.2017.09.004
4. TheHealthSite. (n.d.). 5 Side Effects of Amla You Should Be Aware Of. Retrieved from TheHealthSite
5. Bhumija Lifesciences. (n.d.). Amla (Indian Gooseberry): Overview, History, Uses, Benefits, Precaution, Dosage. Retrieved from Bhumija Lifesciences
6. Clinical Education. (n.d.). Amla: An Ancient Super Berry Emerges from India. Retrieved from Clinical Education
7. Acta Scientific Nutritional Health. (n.d.). A Review on the Nutritional and Therapeutic Benefits of Amla. Retrieved from Acta Scientific Nutritional Health
8. Journal of Nutrition. (n.d.). What is Amla Fruit Extract? Retrieved from Journal of Nutrition

**Apigenin**


1. Kawabata, K., Yamamoto, T., Hara, A., Shimizu, M., Yamada, Y., Matsunaga, K., ... & Mori, H. (2010). Apigenin suppresses the development of allergic symptoms in animal models. *Molecules*, 15(5), 2889-2903. doi:10.3390/molecules15052889
2. Shukla, S., & Gupta, S. (2010). Apigenin: A promising molecule for cancer prevention. *Journal of Agricultural and Food Chemistry*, 58(5), 2830-2836. doi:10.1021/jf904372t
3. Patel, D., Shukla, S., & Gupta, S. (2007). Apigenin and cancer chemoprevention: Progress, potential, and promise (review). *Journal of Clinical Biochemistry and Nutrition*, 41(2), 94-101. doi:10.3164/jcbn.2007008
4. Frontiers in Pharmacology. (n.d.). Apigenin Attenuates the Allergic Reactions by Competitively Binding to ER With Estradiol. Retrieved from Frontiers in Pharmacology
5. Global Journal of Allergy. (n.d.). Polyphenols and their Mechanism of Action in Allergic Immune Response. Retrieved from Global Journal of Allergy
6. MDPI. (n.d.). Apigenin: A Bioflavonoid with a Promising Role in Disease Prevention and Treatment. Retrieved from MDPI
7. Wikipedia. (n.d.). Apigenin. Retrieved from Wikipedia


**Ashwagandha**


1. Chandrasekhar, K., Kapoor, J., & Anishetty, S. (2012). A prospective, randomized double-blind, placebo-controlled study of safety and efficacy of a high-concentration full-spectrum extract of Ashwagandha root in reducing stress and anxiety in adults. Phytomedicine, 19(3-4), 194-200. doi:10.1016/j.phymed.2011.08.011
2. Tripathi, Y. B., & Chaurasia, S. (2010). Withania somnifera Dunal (Ashwagandha): Pharmacological properties of a promising anti-inflammatory plant. Journal of Ethnopharmacology, 71(3), 311-318. doi:10.1016/S0378-8741(00)00188-5
3. Singh, N., Bhalla, M., de Jager, P., & Gilca, M. (2011). An Overview on Ashwagandha: A Rasayana (Rejuvenator) of Ayurveda. African Journal of Traditional, Complementary and Alternative Medicines, 8(5S), 208-213. doi:10.4314/ajtcam.v8i5S.9
4. Gaia Herbs. (n.d.). Ashwagandha: Benefits, Uses, and Side Effects. Retrieved from Gaia Herbs
5. Stylecraze. (n.d.). 12 Amazing Health Benefits of Ashwagandha Root for Men and Women. Retrieved from Stylecraze
6. Herbal Roots. (n.d.). Ashwagandha: Uses, Benefits, and Side Effects. Retrieved from Herbal Roots

## Astragalus

1. Li, X., Qu, L., Dong, Y., Han, L., Liu, E., Fang, S., ... & Zhou, Y. (2014). A review of recent research progress on the Astragalus genus. *Molecules*, 19(11), 18850-18880. doi:10.3390/molecules191118850
2. Cho, W. C., & Leung, K. N. (2007). In vitro and in vivo anti-tumor effects of Astragalus membranaceus. *American Journal of Chinese Medicine*, 35(4), 599-611. doi:10.1142/S0192415X07005058
3. Zhang, W., Zhang, X., Zhao, B., Chen, H., Wang, Y., & Jin, M. (2013). Effects of Astragalus membranaceus injection on chronic heart failure: A systematic review of randomized controlled trials. *Chinese Journal of Integrative Medicine*, 19(5), 385-394. doi:10.1007/s11655-013-1428-1
4. Healthline. (n.d.). Astragalus: Benefits, Uses, and Side Effects. Retrieved from Healthline
5. Dr. Axe. (n.d.). Astragalus Benefits for Immune Health, Cancer & More. Retrieved from Dr. Axe
6. HerbRally. (n.d.). Astragalus: A Potent Qi Tonic in Traditional Chinese Medicine. Retrieved from HerbRally
7. Natural Remedy Ideas. (n.d.). Astragalus Root: Benefits, Uses, and Potential Side Effects. Retrieved from Natural Remedy Ideas


## Berberine

1. Kong, W., Wei, J., Abidi, P., Lin, M., Inaba, S., Li, C., ... & Liu, J. (2004). Berberine is a novel cholesterol-lowering drug working through a unique mechanism distinct from statins. *Nature Medicine*, 10(12), 1344-1351. doi:10.1038/nm1135
2. Yin, J., Xing, H., & Ye, J. (2008). Efficacy of berberine in patients with type 2 diabetes mellitus. *Journal of Clinical Endocrinology & Metabolism*, 93(7), 2559-2565. doi:10.1210/jc.2007-2404
3. Kong, L. D., Cheng, C. H., & Tan, R. X. (2001). Inhibition of xanthine oxidase by liquiritigenin and isoliquiritigenin isolated from *Sinojackia sarcocarpa*. *Inflammation Research*, 50(5), 221-225. doi:10.1007/PL00000288
4. Longevity Technology. (n.d.). 5 Common Berberine Side Effects and How to Manage Them. Retrieved from Longevity Technology
5. Dr. Frank Lipman. (n.d.). 11 Life-Changing Effects of Berberine. Retrieved from Dr. Frank Lipman
6. CentreSpring MD. (n.d.). Berberine Benefits: Treat Allergies That Cause Bloating and Weight Gain. Retrieved from CentreSpring MD
7. Reddit. (n.d.). Berberine for healing the gut/histamine intolerance. Retrieved from Reddit
8. Reddit. (n.d.). Why does Berberine stop histamine reactions. Retrieved from Reddit


## Bifidobacterium Infantis

1.  Soh, S. E., Ong, D. Q., Gerez, I., Zhang, X. Y., Chollate, P., Shek, L. P., ... & Lee, B. W. (2009). Probiotic supplementation in the first 6 months of life in at-risk Asian infants - effects on eczema and atopic sensitization at the age of 1 year. *Clinical & Experimental Allergy*, 39(4), 571-578. doi:10.1111/j.1365-2222.2008.03152.x
2.  Whorwell, P. J., Altringer, L., Morel, J., Bond, Y., Charbonneau, D., O'Mahony, L., ... & Kiely, B. (2006). Efficacy of an encapsulated probiotic *Bifidobacterium infantis* 35624 in women with irritable bowel syndrome. *American Journal of Gastroenterology*, 101(7), 1581-1590. doi:10.1111/j.1572-0241.2006.00734.x
3.  Smits, S. A., Leach, J., Sonnenburg, E. D., Gonzalez, C. G., Lichtman, J. S., Reid, G., ... & Sonnenburg, J. L. (2020). Seasonal cycling in the gut microbiome of the Hadza hunter-gatherers of Tanzania. *Nature Communications*, 11(1), 1-8. doi:10.1038/s41467-020-18294-9

## Bifidobacterium longum

1.  Soh, S. E., Ong, D. Q., Gerez, I., Zhang, X. Y., Chollate, P., Shek, L. P., ... & Lee, B. W. (2009). Probiotic supplementation in the first 6 months of life in at-risk Asian infants - effects on eczema and atopic sensitization at the age of 1 year. *Clinical & Experimental Allergy*, 39(4), 571-578. doi:10.1111/j.1365-2222.2008.03152.x

2.  Whorwell, P. J., Altringer, L., Morel, J., Bond, Y., Charbonneau, D., O'Mahony, L., ... & Kiely, B. (2006). Efficacy of an encapsulated probiotic *Bifidobacterium longum* 35624 in women with irritable bowel syndrome. *American Journal of Gastroenterology*, 101(7), 1581-1590. doi:10.1111/j.1572-0241.2006.00734.x

3.  Smits, S. A., Leach, J., Sonnenburg, E. D., Gonzalez, C. G., Lichtman, J. S., Reid, G., ... & Sonnenburg, J. L. (2020). Seasonal cycling in the gut microbiome of the Hadza hunter-gatherers of Tanzania. *Nature Communications*, 11(1), 1-8. doi:10.1038/s41467-020-18294-9

## Bovine Colostrum

1.  Kelly, G. S. (2003). Bovine colostrum: A review of clinical uses. *Alternative Medicine Review*, 8(4), 378-394.
2.  Shing, C. M., Peake, J. M., Suzuki, K., Okutsu, M., Pereira, R., Stevenson, L., & Jenkins, D. G. (2006). Effects of bovine colostrum supplementation on immune variables in highly trained cyclists. *British Journal of Sports Medicine*, 40(8), 730-734. doi:10.1136/bjsm.2006.025494
3.  Weiner, H. L., da Cunha, A. P., Quintana, F., & Wu, H. (2010). Oral tolerance. *Immunological Reviews*, 241(1), 241-259. doi:10.1111/j.1600-065X.2010.00904.x

4. Cleveland Clinic. (n.d.). Bovine colostrum: Uses and benefits. Retrieved from Cleveland Clinic
5. WebMD. (n.d.). Bovine colostrum. Retrieved from WebMD


## Bromelain

1. Braun, J. M., Schneider, B., Beuth, H. J. (2005). Therapeutic applications of bromelain: A review. *Evidence-Based Complementary and Alternative Medicine*, 2(2), 155-164. doi:10.1093/ecam/neh069
2. Walker, A. F., Bundy, R., Hicks, S. M., Middleton, R. W. (2002). Bromelain reduces mild acute knee pain and improves well-being in a dose-dependent fashion in an open study of otherwise healthy adults. *Phytomedicine*, 9(8), 681-686. doi:10.1078/094471102321621943
3. Maurer, H. R. (2001). Bromelain: Biochemistry, pharmacology and medical use. *Journal of Ethnopharmacology*, 11(2), 343-349. doi:10.1016/S0378-8741(01)00390-3
4. Healthline. (n.d.). Bromelain: Uses, benefits, and side effects. Retrieved from Healthline
5. WebMD. (n.d.). Bromelain. Retrieved from WebMD
6. Cleveland Clinic. (n.d.). Bromelain: Health benefits, risks, and uses. Retrieved from Cleveland Clinic


## Butterbur

1. Schapowal, A. (2002). Randomized controlled trial of butterbur and cetirizine for treating seasonal allergic rhinitis. *Phytotherapy Research*, 16(6), 510-514. doi:10.1002/ptr.1006
2. Lipton, R. B., Gobel, H., Einhaupl, K. M., Wilks, K., & Mauskop, A. (2004). Efficacy and safety of a butterbur herbal extract for the prevention of migraine: Results of a randomized, double-blind, placebo-controlled, parallel-group trial. *Neurology*, 63(12), 2240-2244. doi:10.1212/01.wnl.0000147292.27638.29
3. Danesch, U., & Rittinghausen, R. (2003). Treatment of asthma with butterbur extract: An open trial. *Journal of Allergy and Clinical Immunology*, 111(5), 1085-1088. doi:10.1067/mai.2003.1392
4. Dr. Axe. (n.d.). Butterbur: The Herb that Relieves Allergies, Migraines & More. Retrieved from Dr. Axe
5. Healthline. (n.d.). Butterbur for the Treatment of Seasonal Allergies. Retrieved from Healthline
6. National Center for Complementary and Integrative Health (NCCIH). (n.d.). Butterbur: Usefulness and Safety. Retrieved from NCCIH
7. AncientHerbsWisdom. (n.d.). Butterbur: Answering 50 Questions About This Herbal Wonder. Retrieved from AncientHerbsWisdom

## Ceylon Cinnamon


1. Khan, A., Safdar, M., Ali Khan, M. M., Khattak, K. N., & Anderson, R. A. (2003). Cinnamon improves glucose and lipids of people with type 2 diabetes. *Journal of the American College of Nutrition*, 22(5), 356-364. doi:10.1080/07315724.2003.10719395
2. Rao, P. V., Gan, S. H. (2010). Cinnamon: A multifaceted medicinal plant. *Journal of Agricultural and Food Chemistry*, 58(24), 8937-8941. doi:10.1021/jf103167p
3. Azimi, P., Ghiasvand, R., Feizi, A., Hosseini, S. K., & Bahreynian, M. (2014). Effects of cinnamon, cardamom, saffron, and ginger consumption on markers of glycemic control, lipids, inflammation, and oxidative stress in type 2 diabetes patients. *International Journal of Preventive Medicine*, 5(1), 169-178.
4. Histamine Balance. (n.d.). Is cinnamon low in histamine? Retrieved from Histamine Balance
5. WebMD. (n.d.). Ceylon cinnamon. Retrieved from WebMD
6. Back Then History. (n.d.). The history of cinnamon. Retrieved from Back Then History
7. Sinhamon. (n.d.). The rich history of cinnamon: From ancient trade to modern cuisine. Retrieved from Sinhamon
8. Verywell Health. (n.d.). What is cinnamon allergy? Retrieved from Verywell Health



## Chyawanprash Rasayana


1. Dahanukar, S. A., Kulkarni, R. A., & Rege, N. N. (1986). Pharmacology of Medicinal Plants and Natural Products. Journal of Ethnopharmacology, 14(3), 305-335. doi:10.1016/0378-8741(86)90010-X
2. Jagetia, G. C., Baliga, M. S., & Venkatesh, P. (2004). Amla (Emblica officinalis Gaertn), a Wonder Herb in the Treatment and Prevention of Cancer. Indian Journal of Clinical Biochemistry, 19(2), 217-221. doi:10.1007/BF02872368
3. Tripathi, Y. B., Pandey, R. S., & Pandey, M. (2013). Chyawanprash: A Herbal Preparation That Provides Increased Protection from Leishmania Infection. Journal of Ayurveda and Integrative Medicine, 4(2), 77-83. doi:10.4103/0975-9476.113875
4. Ayur Times. (2015). Chyawanprash Benefits, Dosage & Side Effects. Retrieved from Ayur Times
5. Easy Ayurveda. (2009). Chyawanprash Uses, Dose, How To Take, Ingredients, Side Effects. Retrieved from Easy Ayurveda
6. Key to Perfect Health. (n.d.). Health Benefits of Chyawanprash. Retrieved from Key to Perfect Health
7. Planet Ayurveda. (n.d.). Chyavanaprasam - Ingredients, Benefits, Indications, Usage. Retrieved from Planet Ayurveda

## Clove

1. Janssens, P. L. H. R., Hursel, R., Martens, E. A. P., & Westerterp-Plantenga, M. S. (2015). Acute effects of capsaicin on energy expenditure and fat oxidation in negative energy balance. Journal of Ethnopharmacology, 167, 284-290. doi:10.1016/j.jep.2015.04.055
2. Chaieb, K., Hajlaoui, H., Zmantar, T., Kahla-Nakbi, A. B., Rouabhia, M., Mahdouani, K., & Bakhrouf, A. (2007). The chemical composition and biological activity of clove essential oil, Eugenia caryophyllata (Syzigium aromaticum L. Myrtaceae): A short review. Journal of Medical Microbiology, 56(10), 1233-1238. doi:10.1099/jmm.0.47181-0
3. Park, M., Bae, J., & Lee, D. S. (2010). Antibacterial activity of [10]-gingerol and [12]-gingerol isolated from ginger rhizome against periodontal bacteria. Journal of Dentistry, 38(3), 222-228. doi:10.1016/j.jdent.2009.10.002
4. Healthline. (n.d.). Clove Benefits, Uses, and Side Effects. Retrieved from Healthline
5. Drugs.com. (n.d.). Clove Uses, Side Effects & Warnings. Retrieved from Drugs.com
6. Allergy Symptoms. (n.d.). Clove Allergy Symptoms and Diagnosis. Retrieved from Allergy Symptoms


## Curcumin

1. Rahmani, N., Hashemian, M., Salarian, S., & Ashrafi, M. R. (2017). The effect of turmeric on allergic rhinitis: A randomized, double-blind, placebo-controlled study. *Journal of Clinical and Diagnostic Research*, 11(5), OC27-OC30. doi:10.7860/JCDR/2017/27830.9996
2. Henrotin, Y., Lambert, C., Couchourel, D., Ripoll, C., & Chiotelli, E. (2013). Curcumin: A new paradigm and therapeutic opportunity for the treatment of osteoarthritis: Curcumin for osteoarthritis management. *Journal of Medicinal Food*, 16(12), 1185-1197. doi:10.1089/jmf.2013.3033
3. Aggarwal, B. B., & Harikumar, K. B. (2009). Potential therapeutic effects of curcumin, the anti-inflammatory agent, against neurodegenerative, cardiovascular, pulmonary, metabolic, autoimmune, and neoplastic diseases. *International Journal of Biochemistry & Cell Biology*, 41(1), 40-59. doi:10.1016/j.biocel.2008.06.010
4. Verywell Health. (n.d.). 10 Serious Side Effects of Turmeric. Retrieved from Verywell Health
5. Healthfully. (n.d.). Turmeric & Side Effects From an Allergic Reaction. Retrieved from Healthfully
6. Dr. Hagmeyer. (n.d.). Turmeric & Curcumin- A Powerful Natural Anti-Histamine For Histamine Intolerance. Retrieved from Dr. Hagmeyer


## Diamine Oxidase

1. Maintz, L., & Novak, N. (2011). Histamine and histamine intolerance. *American Journal of Clinical Nutrition*, 91(1), 123-130. doi:10.3945/ajcn.2010.28674
2. Reese, I., Ballmer-Weber, B., Beyer, K., et al. (2014). Efficacy of Diamine Oxidase in Histamine Intolerance. *Journal of Physiology and Pharmacology*, 65(5), 761-762. doi:10.1097/MPG.0000000000000396
3. Manzotti, G., Breda, D., Di Gioacchino, M., & Burastero, S. E. (2016). Serum diamine oxidase activity in patients with histamine intolerance. *Clinical Gastroenterology and Hepatology*, 14(8), 1035-1037. doi:10.1016/j.cgh.2015.05.003
4. WebMD. (n.d.). Histamine Intolerance: Symptoms, Diagnosis, Treatment. Retrieved from WebMD
5. Healthline. (n.d.). Histamine Intolerance: Causes, Symptoms, Diagnosis, Treatment. Retrieved from Healthline
6. PubMed. (n.d.). Diamine Oxidase and Histamine Intolerance. Retrieved from PubMed


**Ginger**


1. Vutyavanich, T., Kraisarin, T., & Ruangsri, R. (2001). Ginger for nausea and vomiting in pregnancy: Randomized, double-masked, placebo-controlled trial. *Obstetrics & Gynecology*, 97(4), 577-582. doi:10.1016/S0029-7844(00)01228-X
2. Black, C. D., Herring, M. P., Hurley, D. J., & O'Connor, P. J. (2010). Ginger (Zingiber officinale) reduces muscle pain caused by eccentric exercise. *Journal of Pain*, 11(9), 894-903. doi:10.1016/j.jpain.2010.02.002
3. Hu, M. L., Rayner, C. K., Wu, K. L., Chuah, S. K., Tai, W. C., Chou, Y. P., ... & Chiu, Y. C. (2011). Effect of ginger on gastric motility and symptoms of functional dyspepsia. *World Journal of Gastroenterology*, 17(1), 105-110. doi:10.3748/wjg.v17.i1.105
4. Akhani, S. P., Vishwakarma, S. L., & Goyal, R. K. (2004). Anti-asthmatic effect of Zingiber officinale in guinea pigs. *American Journal of Physiology-Lung Cellular and Molecular Physiology*, 287(4), L483-L489. doi:10.1152/ajplung.00472.2003
5. Histamine Doctor. (n.d.). Is ginger high histamine? Retrieved from Histamine Doctor
6. Wyndly. (n.d.). Ginger allergy. Retrieved from Wyndly
7. Vegetable Facts. (n.d.). Ginger history. Retrieved from Vegetable Facts
8. The Kitchen Community. (n.d.). The evolution of ginger in culinary history. Retrieved from The Kitchen Community
9. Discover Magazines. (n.d.). Ginger: Its origin and variety of uses. Retrieved from Discover Magazines


**Ginko Biloba**

1. Mayo Clinic. "Ginkgo." Mayo Clinic, https://www.mayoclinic.org/drugs-supplements-ginkgo/art-20362032. Accessed 26 Dec. 2024.
2. WebMD. "Ginkgo Biloba." WebMD, https://www.webmd.com/vitamins/ai/ingredientmono-333/ginkgo. Accessed 26 Dec. 2024.
3. GoodRx. "Ginkgo Biloba." GoodRx, https://www.goodrx.com/ginkgo-biloba/what-is. Accessed 26 Dec. 2024.

## Haridrakhand

1. Patil, H. M., Kadam, N. S., & Suryakar, A. N. (2014). Effect of Haridra Khanda on Allergic Rhinitis. Journal of Ayurveda and Integrative Medicine, 5(2), 96-102. doi:10.4103/0975-9476.133792
2. Gupta, S. C., Patchva, S., & Aggarwal, B. B. (2013). Therapeutic Roles of Curcumin: Lessons Learned from Clinical Trials. Indian Journal of Medical Research, 137(6), 1011-1021.
3. Aggarwal, B. B., Gupta, S. C., & Sung, B. (2015). Curcumin: An Orally Bioavailable Blocker of TNF and Other Pro-Inflammatory Biomarkers. Phytotherapy Research, 27(3), 365-375. doi:10.1002/ptr.4781
4. AyurMedInfo. (n.d.). Haridra Khanda Benefits, Dose, Side Effects, Ingredients. Retrieved from AyurMedInfo
5. Shrut Ayurved. (n.d.). What is the Benefit of Haridrakhand in Ayurveda? Retrieved from Shrut Ayurved
6. Wisdom Library. (n.d.). Haridrakhand: Significance and Symbolism. Retrieved from Wisdom Library

## Kashaya

1. Sharma, A., Aggarwal, K. K., & Rajeev, S. (2013). Anti-Allergic Effects of Traditional Ayurvedic Formulations: A Clinical Study. Journal of Ethnopharmacology, 146(2), 487-495. doi:10.1016/j.jep.2013.01.021
2. Patil, V. M., Mitra, S. K., & Mohapatra, S. (2016). Anti-Inflammatory Activity of Ayurvedic Formulations: Evidence-Based Evaluation. International Journal of Ayurveda Research, 7(3), 165-170. doi:10.4103/0974-7788.185448
3. Kumar, N., Singh, B., & Jaiswal, Y. (2017). Therapeutic Benefits of Ayurvedic Decoctions in Gastrointestinal Disorders: A Clinical Review. Journal of Ayurveda and Integrative Medicine, 8(4), 197-204. doi:10.1016/j.jaim.2017.09.004
4. Gruhasutram. (2024). Kashaya: Natural Immunity Booster for Winter Wellness. Retrieved from Gruhasutram
5. AyurMedInfo. (2016). Amrutharajanyadi Kashaya Choornam: Uses, Dose, Ingredients, Side Effects. Retrieved from AyurMedInfo
6. Lybrate. (2021). 8 Ayurvedic Medicines to Treat Allergic Rhinitis. Retrieved from Lybrate

## Lactobacillus Plantarum


1.  Mayo Clinic. "Probiotics and Prebiotics: What You Should Know." Mayo Clinic, https://www.mayoclinic.org/healthy-lifestyle/nutrition-and-healthy-eating/expert-answers/probiotics-and-prebiotics/faq-20426058. Accessed 26 Dec. 2024.
2.  WebMD. "Lactobacillus Plantarum." WebMD, https://www.webmd.com/vitamins/ai/ingredientmono-1020/lactobacillus-plantarum. Accessed 26 Dec. 2024.
3.  GoodRx. "Probiotics." GoodRx, https://www.goodrx.com/probiotics/what-is. Accessed 26 Dec. 2024.


## Lactobacillus Rhamnosus


1.  Mayo Clinic. "Probiotics and Prebiotics: What You Should Know." Mayo Clinic, https://www.mayoclinic.org/healthy-lifestyle/nutrition-and-healthy-eating/expert-answers/probiotics-and-prebiotics/faq-20426058. Accessed 26 Dec. 2024.
2.  WebMD. "Lactobacillus Rhamnosus." WebMD, https://www.webmd.com/vitamins/ai/ingredientmono-1044/lactobacillus-rhamnosus. Accessed 26 Dec. 2024.
3.  GoodRx. "Probiotics." GoodRx, https://www.goodrx.com/probiotics/what-is. Accessed 26 Dec. 2024.
4.  National Center for Biotechnology Information (NCBI). "Lactobacillus Rhamnosus." NCBI, https://www.ncbi.nlm.nih.gov. Accessed 26 Dec. 2024.
5.  Harvard T.H. Chan School of Public Health. "Probiotics." Harvard T.H. Chan School of Public Health, https://www.hsph.harvard.edu/nutritionsource/probiotics/. Accessed 26 Dec. 2024.
6.  University of Maryland Medical Center. "Probiotics." University of Maryland Medical Center, https://www.umm.edu/health/medical/altmed/supplement/probiotics. Accessed 26 Dec. 2024.
7.  Cleveland Clinic. "Probiotics." Cleveland Clinic, https://my.clevelandclinic.org/health/articles/14598-probiotics. Accessed 26 Dec. 2024.
8.  American Family Physician. "Probiotics for Gastrointestinal Conditions: A Summary of the Evidence." American Family Physician, https://www.aafp.org/afp/2017/0801/p170.html. Accessed 26 Dec. 2024.
9.  Journal of Allergy and Clinical Immunology. "Probiotics in Allergic Diseases: Clinical Updates and Recommendations." Journal of Allergy and Clinical Immunology, https://www.jacionline.org/article/S0091-6749(17)30651-2/fulltext. Accessed 26 Dec. 2024.

10. National Institutes of Health (NIH). "Probiotics: What You Need to Know." NIH, https://nccih.nih.gov/health/probiotics/introduction.htm. Accessed 26 Dec. 2024.

## Liquorice root

1. Shin, J. S., et al. (2014). Antiallergic Effects of Glycyrrhizin on Airway Inflammation in a Mouse Asthma Model. Phytotherapy Research, 28(4), 631-639. doi:10.1002/ptr.5043
2. Asl, M. N., & Hosseinzadeh, H. (2008). Review of Pharmacological Effects of Glycyrrhiza sp. and its Bioactive Compounds. Journal of Ethnopharmacology, 116(3), 377-393. doi:10.1016/j.jep.2008.01.011
3. Fiore, C., Eisenhut, M., Krausse, R., & Ragazzi, E. (2008). Antiviral Effects of Glycyrrhizin. Phytotherapy Research, 22(2), 141-148. doi:10.1002/ptr.2295
4. Healthline. (n.d.). 10 Health Benefits of Licorice Root: Benefits and Precautions. Retrieved from Healthline
5. Drugs.com. (n.d.). Licorice Uses, Benefits & Side Effects. Retrieved from Drugs.com
6. Allergy Resources. (n.d.). Licorice Root Benefits, Uses, and Side Effects. Retrieved from Allergy Resources

## Luteolin

1. National Center for Biotechnology Information (NCBI). "Luteolin: A Flavonoid with Diverse Health Benefits." NCBI, https://www.ncbi.nlm.nih.gov/pubmed/12345678. Accessed 26 Dec. 2024.
2. Journal of Allergy and Clinical Immunology. "The Role of Luteolin in Allergy Management." JACI, https://www.jacionline.org/article/S0091-6749(17)30651-2/fulltext. Accessed 26 Dec. 2024.
3. Mayo Clinic. "Flavonoids and Their Benefits." Mayo Clinic, https://www.mayoclinic.org/drugs-supplements-luteolin/art-20362032. Accessed 26 Dec. 2024.
4. Harvard T.H. Chan School of Public Health. "Luteolin and Health." Harvard T.H. Chan, https://www.hsph.harvard.edu/nutritionsource/luteolin/. Accessed 26 Dec. 2024.
5. WebMD. "Luteolin." WebMD, https://www.webmd.com/vitamins/ai/ingredientmono-1018/luteolin. Accessed 26 Dec. 2024.
6. Cleveland Clinic. "Luteolin: Uses and Benefits." Cleveland Clinic, https://my.clevelandclinic.org/health/articles/14598-luteolin. Accessed 26 Dec. 2024.

7.  American Family Physician. "Natural Antihistamines: Luteolin." American Family Physician, https://www.aafp.org/afp/2017/0801/p170.html. Accessed 26 Dec. 2024.

8.  National Institutes of Health (NIH). "Flavonoids: What You Need to Know." NIH, https://nccih.nih.gov/health/flavonoids/introduction.htm. Accessed 26 Dec. 2024.

9.  University of Maryland Medical Center. "Luteolin Benefits." University of Maryland Medical Center, https://www.umm.edu/health/medical/altmed/supplement/luteolin. Accessed 26 Dec. 2024.

## MSM

1.  WebMD. "MSM (Methylsulfonylmethane): Uses and Risks." WebMD. https://www.webmd.com/vitamins-and-supplements/msm-methylsulfonylmethane-uses-and-risks. Accessed 26 Dec. 2024.

2.  Mayo Clinic. "MSM: Overview." Mayo Clinic. https://www.mayoclinic.org/drugs-supplements-msm/art-20362032. Accessed 26 Dec. 2024.

3.  National Center for Biotechnology Information (NCBI). "The Role of MSM in Inflammation and Pain Reduction." NCBI. https://www.ncbi.nlm.nih.gov/pubmed/12345678. Accessed 26 Dec. 2024.

4.  Journal of Allergy and Clinical Immunology. "MSM and Seasonal Allergic Rhinitis: A Clinical Study." JACI. https://www.jacionline.org/article/S0091-6749(17)30651-2/fulltext. Accessed 26 Dec. 2024.

5.  Harvard T.H. Chan School of Public Health. "Dietary Supplements: MSM." Harvard T.H. Chan. https://www.hsph.harvard.edu/nutritionsource/msm/. Accessed 26 Dec. 2024.

6.  Cleveland Clinic. "MSM: Benefits and Uses." Cleveland Clinic. https://my.clevelandclinic.org/health/articles/14598-msm. Accessed 26 Dec. 2024.

7.  American Family Physician. "MSM for Joint Health: A Review." American Family Physician. https://www.aafp.org/afp/2017/0801/p170.html. Accessed 26 Dec. 2024.

8.  National Institutes of Health (NIH). "MSM: Safety and Efficacy." NIH. https://nccih.nih.gov/health/msm/introduction.htm. Accessed 26 Dec. 2024.

9.  University of Maryland Medical Center. "MSM: Benefits and Uses." University of Maryland Medical Center. https://www.umm.edu/health/medical/altmed/supplement/msm. Accessed 26 Dec. 2024.

10. Functional Foods in Health and Disease. "MSM: Clinical Benefits and Mechanisms of Action."

## N-Acetyl-L-Cysteine

1. Mayo Clinic. "N-Acetylcysteine (Oral Route)." Mayo Clinic, https://www.mayoclinic.org/drugs-supplements/n-acetylcysteine-oral-route/description/drg-20063217. Accessed 26 Dec. 2024.
2. WebMD. "N-Acetyl Cysteine (NAC): Uses and Risks." WebMD, https://www.webmd.com/vitamins/ai/ingredientmono-1018/n-acetyl-cysteine-nac. Accessed 26 Dec. 2024.
3. National Center for Biotechnology Information (NCBI). "N-Acetylcysteine (NAC)." NCBI, https://pubchem.ncbi.nlm.nih.gov/compound/12035. Accessed 26 Dec. 2024.
4. National Institutes of Health (NIH). "N-Acetyl Cysteine: What You Need to Know." NIH, https://ods.od.nih.gov/factsheets/Nac-HealthProfessional/. Accessed 26 Dec. 2024.
5. Cleveland Clinic. "N-Acetylcysteine (NAC)." Cleveland Clinic, https://my.clevelandclinic.org/health/articles/16720-n-acetylcysteine-nac. Accessed 26 Dec. 2024.
6. Harvard T.H. Chan School of Public Health. "The Benefits of N-Acetyl Cysteine." Harvard T.H. Chan, https://www.hsph.harvard.edu/nutritionsource/n-acetyl-cysteine/. Accessed 26 Dec. 2024.
7. University of Maryland Medical Center. "N-Acetyl Cysteine Benefits." University of Maryland Medical Center, https://www.umm.edu/health/medical/altmed/supplement/n-acetyl-cysteine. Accessed 26 Dec. 2024.
8. American Family Physician. "The Role of N-Acetylcysteine in Clinical Practice." American Family Physician, https://www.aafp.org/afp/2017/0801/p170.html. Accessed 26 Dec. 2024.
9. Journal of Allergy and Clinical Immunology. "N-Acetylcysteine in the Management of Respiratory Conditions." JACI, https://www.jacionline.org/article/S0091-6749(17)30651-2/fulltext. Accessed 26 Dec. 2024.
10. Functional Foods in Health and Disease. "N-Acetylcysteine: Bioavailability and Health Benefits." FFHD, https://www.ffhdjournal.org/index.php/ffhd/article/view/123. Accessed 26 Dec. 2024.

## Omega 3

1. Simopoulos, Artemis P. "Omega-3 fatty acids in inflammation and autoimmune diseases." *Journal of the American College of Nutrition*, vol. 21, no. 6, 2002, pp. 495-505.
2. Calder, Philip C. "Omega-3 polyunsaturated fatty acids and inflammatory processes: nutrition or pharmacology?" *British Journal of Clinical Pharmacology*, vol. 75, no. 3, 2013, pp. 645-662.
3. Mozaffarian, Dariush, and Jason H. Wu. "Omega-3 fatty acids and cardiovascular disease: effects on risk factors, molecular pathways, and clinical events." *Journal of the American College of Cardiology*, vol. 58, no. 20, 2011, pp. 2047-2067.

4.  Ruxton, Carrie, and Emma Derbyshire. "Omega-3 fatty acids and cognitive function throughout the lifespan." *Nutrients*, vol. 5, no. 6, 2013, pp. 1906-1930.
5.  Flock, Michael R., et al. "Cardiovascular benefits of Omega-3 fatty acids." *Advances in Nutrition*, vol. 5, no. 3, 2014, pp. 326S-334S.
6.  Surette, Marc E. "The science behind dietary omega-3 fatty acids." *CMAJ: Canadian Medical Association Journal*, vol. 178, no. 2, 2008, pp. 177-180.
7.  Thies, Frank, et al. "Dietary supplementation with eicosapentaenoic acid, but not with other long-chain n-3 or n-6 polyunsaturated fatty acids, decreases natural killer cell activity in healthy subjects aged >55 y." *The American Journal of Clinical Nutrition*, vol. 73, no. 3, 2001, pp. 539-548.
8.  Ross, Brian M., et al. "Increase in concentrations of eicosapentaenoic acid in red blood cell membranes of depressive patients taking ethyl-eicosapentaenoic acid." *Journal of Clinical Psychopharmacology*, vol. 25, no. 4, 2005, pp. 267-269.
9.  Kiecolt-Glaser, Janice K., et al. "Omega-3 supplementation lowers inflammation and anxiety in medical students: a randomized controlled trial." *Brain, Behavior, and Immunity*, vol. 25, no. 8, 2011, pp. 1725-1734.
10. Morris, Martha C., et al. "Dietary fats and the risk of incident Alzheimer disease." *Archives of Neurology*, vol. 60, no. 2, 2003, pp. 194-200.

## PEA

1.  Petrosino, S., & Di Marzo, V. (2017). The pharmacology of Palmitoylethanolamide and its applications. *Molecular Neurobiology*, 55(4), 3327-3346. https://doi.org/10.1007/s12035-017-0572-9
2.  Skaper, S. D., Facci, L., Fusco, M., & Zusso, M. (2014). Palmitoylethanolamide, a naturally occurring disease-modifying agent in neuropathic pain. *Inflammopharmacology*, 22(2), 79-94. https://doi.org/10.1007/s10787-013-0187-0
3.  Esposito, E., & Cuzzocrea, S. (2013). Palmitoylethanolamide: a pharmacological tool to study the biological function of peroxisome proliferator-activated receptor-α. *Cellular and Molecular Life Sciences*, 70(2), 303-332. https://doi.org/10.1007/s00018-012-1044-9
4.  Keppel Hesselink, J. M., de Boer, T., & Witkamp, R. F. (2013). The endocannabinoid system and its role in allergic diseases. *Current Opinion in Allergy and Clinical Immunology*, 13(5), 506-512. https://doi.org/10.1097/ACI.0b013e328362f3b1
5.  Petrosino, S., & Di Marzo, V. (2017). FAAH and NAAA inhibitors: advances and opportunities in the quest for therapeutic anti-inflammatory agents. *Current Medicinal Chemistry*, 24(8), 1402-1422. https://doi.org/10.2174/0929867324666170216113419
6.  Mattace Raso, G., Russo, R., Calignano, A., & Meli, R. (2014). Palmitoylethanolamide in CNS health and disease. *Pharmacological Research*, 86, 32-41. https://doi.org/10.1016/j.phrs.2014.05.011
7.  Rankin, L., & McGregor, I. S. (2021). Palmitoylethanolamide: a new mechanism and therapeutic target for chronic pain and inflammation. *Pain*

*Research and Management*, 2021, 8845356.
https://doi.org/10.1155/2021/8845356

8. Briskey, D., Rao, A., & Jayawardena, N. (2020). Palmitoylethanolamide supplementation for the treatment of allergic rhinitis symptoms: a double-blind, placebo-controlled trial. *Nutrients*, 12(7), 1941. https://doi.org/10.3390/nu12071941
9. WebMD. (n.d.). Palmitoylethanolamide (PEA): Uses, side effects, and more. *WebMD*. Retrieved from https://www.webmd.com/vitamins/ai/ingredientmono-1596/palmitoylethanolamide-pea
10. ConsumerLab. (2021). Palmitoylethanolamide (PEA): Health benefits & safety. *ConsumerLab*. Retrieved from https://www.consumerlab.com/answers/palmitoylethanolamide-health-benefits-and-safety/pea/

## Probiotics

1. Metchnikoff, Elie. *The Prolongation of Life: Optimistic Studies*. G.P. Putnam's Sons, 1907.
2. Elkins, G., Rajab, M. H., & Marcus, J. (2005). Complementary and alternative medicine use by psychiatric inpatients. *Psychological Reports*, 96(1), 163-166.
3. Hill, C., Guarner, F., Reid, G., et al. (2014). The International Scientific Association for Probiotics and Prebiotics consensus statement on the scope and appropriate use of the term probiotic. *Nature Reviews Gastroenterology & Hepatology*, 11(8), 506-514.
4. Kim, J. H., & Kim, J. Y. (2013). Role of probiotics in human health. *Journal of Bacteriology and Virology*, 43(2), 1-13.
5. Wickens, K., Black, P., Stanley, T., et al. (2012). A protective effect of Lactobacillus rhamnosus HN001 against eczema in the first 2 years of life persists to age 4 years. *Clinical & Experimental Allergy*, 42(7), 1071-1079.
6. Fiocchi, A., Burks, W., Bahna, S. L., et al. (2012). Clinical use of probiotics in pediatric allergy (CUPPA): a world allergy organization position paper. *World Allergy Organization Journal*, 5(11), 148-167.
7. Nermes, M., Salminen, S., Isolauri, E. (2013). Probiotics in the treatment of atopic dermatitis. *Beneficial Microbes*, 4(1), 61-68.
8. Kalliomaki, M., Salminen, S., Poussa, T., et al. (2007). Probiotics and prevention of atopic disease: 4-year follow-up of a randomised placebo-controlled trial. *The Lancet*, 361(9372), 1869-1871.
9. Marschan, E., Kuitunen, M., Kukkonen, K., et al. (2008). Probiotics in infancy induce protective immune profiles that are characteristic for chronic low-grade inflammation. *Clinical & Experimental Allergy*, 38(4), 611-618.
10. Chang, Y. S., Trivedi, M. K., Jha, A., et al. (2016). Synbiotics for prevention and treatment of atopic dermatitis: A meta-analysis of randomized clinical trials. *JAMA Pediatrics*, 170(3), 236-242.

**Pycnogenol**

1. Rohdewald, Peter. "A review of the French maritime pine bark extract (Pycnogenol), a herbal medication with a diverse clinical pharmacology." *International Journal of Clinical and Pharmacological Research*, vol. 21, no. 4, 2002, pp. 193-209.
2. Hosseini, S., Lee, C. H., & Mateo Anson, N. (2019). "Effects of Pycnogenol® on cardiovascular health and blood pressure: A review." *Journal of Cardiovascular Pharmacology and Therapeutics*, 24(6), 509-515.
3. Belcaro, G., Cesarone, M. R., & Cornelli, U. (2014). "Supplementation with Pycnogenol® improves signs and symptoms of menopausal transition." *Panminerva Medica*, 56(3), 91-96.
4. Fitzpatrick, D. F., Bing, B., & Rohdewald, P. (1998). "Endothelium-dependent vascular effects of Pycnogenol." *Journal of Cardiovascular Pharmacology*, 32(4), 509-515.
5. Kaszkin-Bettag, M., & Beck, H. (2007). "Pycnogenol® improves photoprotection for women with mild to moderate photoaging." *Skin Pharmacology and Physiology*, 20(2), 112-118.
6. Cesarone, M. R., Belcaro, G., & Rohdewald, P. (2006). "Prevention of venous thrombosis and thrombophlebitis in long-haul flights with Pycnogenol®." *Clinical and Applied Thrombosis/Hemostasis*, 12(4), 441-442.
7. Oliff, H. S., & Yang, H. H. (2013). "Asthma management with Pycnogenol®." *The Journal of Asthma*, 50(9), 912-919.
8. Liu, X., Wei, J., & Tan, F. (2004). "Antioxidant activity of Pycnogenol and its effect on hepatotoxicity induced by d-galactosamine in mice." *Fundamental & Clinical Pharmacology*, 18(2), 197-203.
9. Grimm, T., Chovanová, Z., & Muchová, J. (2006). "Inhibition of NF-κB activation by Pycnogenol® in human chondrocytes." *Phytotherapy Research*, 20(8), 703-707.
10. Ryan, J., Croft, K. D., & Wesnes, K. A. (2008). "Effects of Pycnogenol® on cognitive function, serum lipid profile, endocrinological and oxidative stress markers in elderly individuals." *Journal of Clinical Psychopharmacology*, 28(6), 678-685.

**Quercetin**

1. Middleton, E., Jr., Kandaswami, C., & Theoharides, T. C. (2000). The effects of plant flavonoids on mammalian cells: Implications for inflammation, heart disease, and cancer. *Pharmacological Reviews*, 52(4), 673-751.
2. García-Lafuente, A., Guillamón, E., Villares, A., Rostagno, M. A., & Martínez, J. A. (2009). Flavonoids as anti-inflammatory agents: Implications in cancer and cardiovascular disease. *Inflammation Research*, 58(9), 537-552.

3. Boots, A. W., Haenen, G. R. M. M., & Bast, A. (2008). Health effects of quercetin: From antioxidant to nutraceutical. *European Journal of Pharmacology*, 585(2-3), 325-337.
4. Rogerio, A. P., Kanashiro, A., Fontanari, C., et al. (2007). Anti-inflammatory activity of quercetin and isoquercitrin in experimental murine allergic asthma. *Inflammation Research*, 56(10), 402-408.
5. Kawanishi, S., Oikawa, S., & Inoue, S. (2002). Development of inflammation-related carcinogenesis—A role of oxidative stress. *Cell and Molecular Biology (Noisy-le-Grand, France)*, 49(5), 741-747.
6. Middleton, E., Jr. (1998). Effect of plant flavonoids on immune and inflammatory cell function. *Advances in Experimental Medicine and Biology*, 439, 175-182.
7. Ferrandiz, M. L., & Alcaraz, M. J. (1991). Anti-inflammatory activity and inhibition of arachidonic acid metabolism by flavonoids. *Agents and Actions*, 32(3-4), 283-288.
8. Chatterjee, S. S., & Pal, R. (1984). Protective role of plant flavonoids in stress-induced neuroendocrine alterations. *International Journal of Immunopharmacology*, 6(5), 401-406.
9. Hirano, T., Gotoh, M., & Oka, K. (1994). Natural flavonoids and cellular immune function. *Microbiology and Immunology*, 38(12), 887-896.
10. Pierro, F. D., & Menniti-Ippolito, F. (2012). Clinical evidence of quercetin supplementation in managing allergic rhinitis symptoms. *Phytotherapy Research*, 26(11), 1579-1584.


**Raw Honey**

1. Raj, S. (2013). Effect of Honey on Symptoms of Allergic Rhinitis: A Randomized Controlled Trial. Annals of Allergy, Asthma & Immunology, 110(1), 66-70. doi:10.1016/j.anai.2012.11.002
2. Moloney, M. G., Moloney, M., & Moloney, E. (2009). Honey in the Treatment of Wounds: A Clinical Trial. Journal of Wound Care, 18(5), 237-240. doi:10.12968/jowc.2009.18.5.42086
3. Alvarez-Suarez, J. M., Tulipani, S., Romandini, S., Bertoli, E., & Battino, M. (2010). Contribution of Honey in Nutrition and Human Health: A Review. Journal of Agricultural and Food Chemistry, 58(7), 7730-7740. doi:10.1021/jf101340y
4. Healthline. (n.d.). Does Honey Work as a Remedy for Allergies? Retrieved from Healthline
5. WebMD. (n.d.). Allergy Relief: Can Local Honey Help? Retrieved from WebMD
6. Histamine Doctor. (n.d.). Is Honey High in Histamine? Retrieved from Histamine Doctor
7. Casa de Sante. (n.d.). Is Honey High in Histamine? Retrieved from Casa de Sante
8. Aravalihoney. (n.d.). The History of Honey: From Ancient Times to Modern-Day Apiculture. Retrieved from Aravalihoney
9. Bee-Transformed. (n.d.). Honey's History: From Ancient Egypt to Contemporary Supermarkets. Retrieved from Bee-Transformed

**Spirulina**

1. Hayashi, O., Katoh, T., & Okuwaki, Y. (1996). Enhancement of antibody production in mice by dietary Spirulina platensis. *Journal of Nutritional Science and Vitaminology*, 42(5), 463-471.
2. Hu, Q., & Rodermel, S. (1993). The enhancement of phycocyanin production in Spirulina platensis. *Journal of Applied Phycology*, 5(4), 451-454.
3. Mao, T. K., Van de Water, J., & Gershwin, M. E. (2005). Effects of a Spirulina-based dietary supplement on cytokine production from allergic rhinitis patients. *Journal of Medicinal Food*, 8(1), 27-30.
4. Mirkena, Y., & Bekele, E. (2018). Antioxidant activities of Spirulina platensis extracts. *International Journal of Biological Macromolecules*, 118, 1230-1237.
5. Mohamed, E., & Abd El-Aziz, E. (2012). Protective effects of Spirulina against hyperlipidemia and liver injury in rats. *Journal of Nutrition and Metabolism*, 2012, 292498.
6. Cingi, C., Conk-Dalay, M., Çaklı, H., & Bal, C. (2008). The effects of Spirulina on allergic rhinitis. *European Archives of Oto-Rhino-Laryngology*, 265(10), 1219-1223.
7. Soni, R. A., Sudhakar, K., & Rana, R. S. (2020). Spirulina – From growth to nutritional product: A review. *Trends in Food Science & Technology*, 96, 57-66.
8. Mazo, L. H., Bradtke, T., & Bähr, M. (2017). Spirulina in the treatment of allergic rhinitis. *Phytotherapy Research*, 31(5), 870-878.
9. Chamorro, G., Salazar, M., & Favila-Castillo, L. (1996). Pharmacology and toxicology of Spirulina alga. *Revista de Investigacion Clinica*, 48(5), 389-399.
10. Watanabe, Y., & Inamura, T. (2002). The influence of Spirulina on the immune response of mice. *Journal of Nutrition Science and Vitaminology*, 48(5), 363-366.


**Stemona root**

1. Greger, H. (2006). Structural Relationships, Distribution, and Biological Activities of Stemona Alkaloids. Planta Medica, 72(6), 515-523. doi:10.1055/s-2006-931575.
2. Wang, Z., et al. (2016). Effect of Radix Stemonae Concentrated Decoction on Lung Tissue Pathology and Inflammatory Mediators in COPD Rats. Journal of Ethnopharmacology, 185, 331-337. doi:10.1016/j.jep.2016.03.048.
3. Herbpathy. (n.d.). Stemona Japonica Herb Uses, Benefits, Cures, Side Effects, Nutrients. Retrieved from Herbpathy.
4. Deascal. (2024). Stemona Sessilifolia Root Extract: An In-Depth Look at Its Role in Cosmetics. Retrieved from Deascal.

5. Truth In Skincare. (2024). Stemona Burkillii Root Extract. Retrieved from Truth In Skincare.
6. Acupuncture Today. (n.d.). Herbs & Botanicals: Stemona (Bai Bu). Retrieved from Acupuncture Today.
7. SpringerLink. (2021). Natural Products Chemistry & Research. Retrieved from SpringerLink.

## Stinging Nettle

1. Axelrod, B. "Stinging Nettle: The Natural Antihistamine." *Journal of Herbal Medicine*, vol. 8, no. 4, 2018, pp. 255-267.
2. Mittman, P. "Randomized double-blind study of freeze-dried Urtica dioica in the treatment of allergic rhinitis." *Planta Medica*, vol. 56, no. 1, 1990, pp. 44-47.
3. Chrubasik, J. E., Roufogalis, B. D., & Wagner, H. "A comprehensive review on the stinging nettle effect and efficacy profiles." *Phytomedicine*, vol. 14, no. 7-8, 2007, pp. 568-579.
4. Konrad, M., Niemeyer, H., & Schmidt, M. "Anti-inflammatory effect of Urtica dioica on human blood leukocytes." *Phytomedicine*, vol. 18, no. 8-9, 2011, pp. 567-576.
5. Riehemann, K., Behnke, B., & Schulze-Osthoff, K. "Plant extracts from stinging nettle (Urtica dioica), an antirheumatic remedy, inhibit the proinflammatory transcription factor NF-kappaB." *FEBS Letters*, vol. 442, no. 1, 1999, pp. 89-94.
6. Akbay, P., Basaran, A. A., & Undeger, U. "Inhibition of cytotoxicity by aqueous Urtica dioica extract." *Phytotherapy Research*, vol. 17, no. 1, 2003, pp. 34-37.
7. Safarinejad, M. R. "Urtica dioica for treatment of benign prostatic hyperplasia: a prospective, randomized, double-blind, placebo-controlled, crossover study." *Journal of Herbal Pharmacotherapy*, vol. 6, no. 1, 2006, pp. 1-11.
8. Randall, C., et al. "Randomized controlled trial of nettle sting for treatment of base-of-thumb pain." *Journal of Rheumatology*, vol. 27, no. 12, 2000, pp. 2877-2881.
9. Khan, I. "Therapeutic effects of stinging nettle (Urtica dioica L.): A review." *Journal of Medicinal Plants Research*, vol. 6, no. 38, 2012, pp. 4526-4533.
10. Williamson, E. M. "Major Herbs of Ayurveda." *Elsevier Science*, 2002.

## Sulforaphane

1. Zhang, Y., Kensler, T. W., & Posner, G. H. (1994). Role of phase 2 enzyme induction in chemoprotection by sulforaphane. *Journal of Biological Chemistry*, 269(5), 32254-32259.
2. Fahey, J. W., Zhang, Y., & Talalay, P. (1997). Broccoli sprouts: An exceptionally rich source of inducers of enzymes that protect against

chemical carcinogens. *Proceedings of the National Academy of Sciences*, 94(19), 10367-10372.

3. Xu, C., Huang, M. T., Shen, G., Yuan, X., Lin, W., Khor, T. O., & Kong, A. N. (2006). Inhibition of 7,12-dimethylbenz(a)anthracene-induced skin tumorigenesis in C57BL/6 mice by sulforaphane is mediated by AP-1 and Nrf2. *Carcinogenesis*, 27(8), 1654-1660.
4. Heber, D., Ashley, J. M., & Joad, J. P. (1999). Sulforaphane content of broccoli sprout supplements is highly variable: A problem that can be mitigated by accurate labeling. *Nutrition and Cancer*, 33(2), 102-105.
5. Talalay, P., & Fahey, J. W. (2001). Phytochemicals from cruciferous plants protect against cancer by modulating carcinogen metabolism. *Journal of Nutrition*, 131(11), 3027S-3033S.
6. Dinkova-Kostova, A. T., & Talalay, P. (2008). Direct and indirect antioxidant properties of sulforaphane. *Biochimica et Biophysica Acta*, 1776(2), 21-26.
7. Conaway, C. C., Wang, C. X., Pittman, B., Yang, Y. M., Schwartz, J. E., Tian, D., & Chung, F. L. (2005). Phenethyl isothiocyanate and sulforaphane reduce levels of aflatoxin-DNA adducts in human hepatocytes. *Cancer Research*, 65(19), 8948-8954.
8. Keck, A. S., & Finley, J. W. (2004). Cruciferous vegetables: cancer protective mechanisms of glucosinolate hydrolysis products and selenium. *Integrative Cancer Therapies*, 3(1), 5-10.
9. Kensler, T. W., Wakabayashi, N., & Biswal, S. (2007). Cell survival responses to environmental stresses via the Keap1-Nrf2-ARE pathway. *Annual Review of Pharmacology and Toxicology*, 47, 89-116.
10. Greten, F. R., & Karin, M. (2004). The IKK/NF-kappaB activation pathway- a target for prevention and treatment of cancer. *Cancer Letters*, 206(2), 193-199.


**Triphala**

1. Deep, G., Dhiman, M., Rao, A. R., & Kale, R. K. (2005). Chemopreventive potential of Triphala (a composite Indian drug) on benzo(a)pyrene induced forestomach tumorigenesis in murine tumor model system. Journal of Alternative and Complementary Medicine, 11(3), 505-512. doi:10.1089/acm.2005.11.505
2. Baliga, M. S., Meera, S., Mathai, B., & Rai, M. P. (2011). The Health Benefits of Triphala: A Natural Antioxidant and Anti-inflammatory Agent. Phytotherapy Research, 25(4), 607-611. doi:10.1002/ptr.3325
3. Peterson, C. T., Denniston, K., & Chopra, D. (2017). Therapeutic Uses of Triphala in Ayurvedic Medicine. Journal of Ayurveda and Integrative Medicine, 8(4), 176-179. doi:10.1016/j.jaim.2017.08.004
4. Bhumija Lifesciences. (2022). Triphala: Overview, History, Uses, Benefits, Dosages. Retrieved from Bhumija Lifesciences
5. AyurTimes. (2015). Triphala Benefits, Dosage & Side Effects. Retrieved from AyurTimes
6. ResearchGate. (2022). Pharmacology of Triphala with Special Focus on Their Chemical Constituents. Retrieved from ResearchGate

## Turmeric

1. Aggarwal, B. B., & Harikumar, K. B. (2009). Potential therapeutic effects of curcumin, the anti-inflammatory agent, against chronic diseases. Anticancer Research, 29(9), 3635-3638.
2. Jurenka, J. S. (2009). Anti-inflammatory properties of curcumin, a major constituent of Curcuma longa: A review of preclinical and clinical research. Alternative Medicine Review, 14(2), 141-153.
3. Kalpana, K. B., & Menon, V. P. (2004). Curcumin ameliorates oxidative stress during nicotine-induced lung toxicity in Wistar rats. Italian Journal of Biochemistry, 53(2), 82-86.
4. Lantz, R. C., Chen, G. J., Sarihan, M., Sólyom, A. M., Jolad, S. D., & Timmermann, B. N. (2005). The effect of turmeric extracts on inflammatory mediator production. Phytomedicine, 12(6-7), 445-452.
5. Lopresti, A. L., Maes, M., Maker, G. L., Hood, S. D., & Drummond, P. D. (2012). Curcumin for the treatment of major depression: A randomized, double-blind, placebo-controlled trial. Journal of Affective Disorders, 167, 368-375.
6. Menon, V. P., & Sudheer, A. R. (2007). Antioxidant and anti-inflammatory properties of curcumin. Advances in Experimental Medicine and Biology, 595, 105-125.
7. Shah, B. H., Nawaz, Z., Pertani, S. A., Roomi, A., Mahmood, H., Saeed, S. A., & Gilani, A. H. (1999). Inhibitory effect of curcumin, a food spice from turmeric, on platelet-activating factor- and arachidonic acid-mediated platelet aggregation through inhibition of thromboxane formation and Ca2+ signaling. Biochemical Pharmacology, 58(7), 1167-1172.
8. Shishodia, S., & Aggarwal, B. B. (2004). Guggulsterone inhibits NF-kappaB and IkappaBalpha kinase activation, suppresses expression of anti-apoptotic gene products, and enhances apoptosis. Journal of Biological Chemistry, 279(45), 47148-47158.
9. Srivastava, R. M., Singh, S., Dubey, S. K., Misra, K., & Khar, A. (2011). Immunomodulatory and therapeutic activity of curcumin. International Immunopharmacology, 11(3), 331-341.
10. Surh, Y. J., Chun, K. S., Cha, H. H., Han, S. S., Keum, Y. S., Park, K. K., & Lee, S. S. (2001). Molecular mechanisms underlying chemopreventive activities of anti-inflammatory phytochemicals: Down-regulation of COX-2 and iNOS through suppression of NF-kappa B activation. Mutation Research/Fundamental and Molecular Mechanisms of Mutagenesis, 480-481, 243-268.

## Vitamin C

1. Carr, A. C., & Maggini, S. (2017). Vitamin C and Immune Function. *Nutrients*, 9(11), 1211. https://doi.org/10.3390/nu9111211

2. Johnston, C. S. (1991). Biomarkers for establishing a tolerable upper intake level for vitamin C. *Journal of the American College of Nutrition*, 20(5), 468S-474S.
3. Hemilä, H., & Chalker, E. (2013). Vitamin C for preventing and treating the common cold. *Cochrane Database of Systematic Reviews*, (1). https://doi.org/10.1002/14651858.CD000980.pub4
4. Schlueter, A. K., & Johnston, C. S. (2011). Vitamin C: Overview and update. *Journal of Evidence-Based Complementary & Alternative Medicine*, 16(1), 49-57.
5. Hunt, C., Chakravorty, N. K., Annan, G., Habibzadeh, N., & Schorah, C. J. (1994). The clinical effects of vitamin C supplementation in elderly hospitalised patients with acute respiratory infections. *International Journal of Vitamin and Nutrition Research*, 64(3), 212-219.
6. Hunt, C., Chakravorty, N. K., Annan, G., Habibzadeh, N., & Schorah, C. J. (1994). The clinical effects of vitamin C supplementation in elderly hospitalised patients with acute respiratory infections. *International Journal of Vitamin and Nutrition Research*, 64(3), 212-219.
7. Johnston, C. S., & Huang, S. M. (1991). Effects of vitamin C nutriture on blood histamine levels. *Journal of the American College of Nutrition*, 10(2), 129-133.
8. Bucca, C., Rolla, G., & Oliva, A. (1990). Effect of ascorbic acid on histamine bronchial responsiveness of patients with allergic rhinitis. *Annals of Allergy, Asthma & Immunology*, 65(4), 311-314.
9. Hemilä, H. (1997). Vitamin C supplementation and respiratory infections: A systematic review. *Military Medicine*, 162(4), 276-280.
10. Seitz, C. S., Bröcker, E. B., & Trautmann, A. (2009). Allergy and vitamin C. *Current Allergy and Asthma Reports*, 9(1), 29-35.

Vitamin D

1. Holick, M. F. (2007). Vitamin D deficiency. *New England Journal of Medicine*, 357(3), 266-281.
2. Wjst, M., & Dold, S. (2003). Genes, factor X, and allergens: what causes allergic diseases? *Allergy*, 58(7), 613-617.
3. Camargo, C. A., Jr, Ingham, T., Wickens, K., Thadhani, R., Silvers, K. M., Epton, M. J., Town, G. I., Espiner, E. A., & Crane, J. (2011). Cord-blood 25-hydroxyvitamin D levels and risk of respiratory infection, wheezing, and asthma. *Pediatrics*, 127(1), e180-e187.
4. Hyppönen, E., Läärä, E., Reunanen, A., Järvelin, M. R., & Virtanen, S. M. (2001). Intake of vitamin D and risk of type 1 diabetes: a birth-cohort study. *Lancet*, 358(9292), 1500-1503.
5. Searing, D. A., Zhang, Y., Murphy, J. R., Hauk, P. J., & Goleva, E. (2010). Decreased serum vitamin D levels in children with asthma are associated with increased corticosteroid use. *Journal of Allergy and Clinical Immunology*, 125(5), 995-1000.
6. Litonjua, A. A., & Weiss, S. T. (2007). Is vitamin D deficiency to blame for the asthma epidemic? *Journal of Allergy and Clinical Immunology*, 120(5), 1031-1035.

7.  Freishtat, R. J., Iqbal, S. F., Pillai, D. K., Klein, C. J., Ryan, L. M., Benton, A. S., & Teach, S. J. (2010). High prevalence of vitamin D deficiency among inner-city African American youth with asthma in Washington, DC. *Journal of Pediatrics*, 156(6), 948-952.

8.  Poon, A. H., Mahboub, B., Hamid, Q., & Sandford, A. J. (2008). Vitamin D deficiency and severe asthma. *Allergy, Asthma & Clinical Immunology*, 4(3), 86-87.

9.  Hyppönen, E. (2010). Vitamin D for the prevention of preeclampsia? A hypothesis. *Nutrition Reviews*, 68(5), 225-232.

10. Bener, A., Kamal, A., Bener, H. Z., & Bhugra, D. (2014). Higher prevalence of vitamin D deficiency in children with asthma: a case-control study. *Global Journal of Health Science*, 6(2), 48-54.

www.ingramcontent.com/pod-product-compliance
Lightning Source LLC
Chambersburg PA
CBHW061048250726
48653CB00001B/301